# THE POSTURE WORKBOOK

## Carolyn Nicholls

NG

g.com

First published in 2012 by D & B Publishing

British Library Cataloguing-in-Publication Data
A catalogue record for this book is available from the British Library.

ISBN 978 1 904468 79 0

All sales enquiries should be directed to:
email: info@dandbpublishing.com
website: www.dandbpublishing.com

Cover design by Horacio Monteverde
Produced for D&B Publishing by Posthouse Publishing
Printed and bound in China by 1010 Print International Ltd

"Every singer, musician or actor will have experienced tensions or postural problems at some stage. The Alexander Technique is a successful way of training the body to cope with these strains; and this book is an indispensable 'self-help' addition to the performer's library."

**Neil Jenkins**
**Professional Opera Singer**

"With many of us leading busy and pressured lives we often suffer with neck, back and shoulder pain, not to mention stiffness in our fingers after typing for hours. I have been a fan of the Alexander Technique for most of my adult life as I've found it's a way to help my body to continue to serve me. In her comprehensive self-help Posture Workbook Carolyn Nicholls has managed to convey in simple and understandable terms, supported by excellent graphics, how to consciously command our muscles so that we manage pain and stiffness. Carolyn makes her specially designed postural exercises in her 5-a-day plan as easy to incorporate into our daily lives as cleaning our teeth. Benefitting from the wisdom in the Posture Workbook is a must for any active person who wishes to minimise physical discomfort as a result of everyday living."

**Maryon Stewart**
**Natural Health Expert and TV Presenter**

Reviews for
*Body, Breath and Being: A new guide to the Alexander Technique*
by Carolyn Nicholls

"Fantastic, great pictures, a very informative practical book. This goes on our reading list for BA and MA students".

**Chris Palmer**
**Head of Voice and Speech at GSA School of Acting and Musical Theatre**

"I have had Alexander lessons throughout my career, found them invaluable and recommended them to countless other singers. Congratulations to Carolyn Nicholls, who has distilled her many years of teaching into this lucid, down to earth and entertaining book; it will work well for newcomers and devotees alike (singers and normal folk!), whether as introduction to or reminder of this marvellous technique."

**Dame Emma Kirkby**
**Soprano**

"Carolyn Nicholls' book is much more than a beginner's introduction to the Alexander Technique. Teachers of the technique will also find this book a useful manual for honing their communication skills and expanding their repertoire of handy hints and ideas. Carolyn's expertise as a teacher shows through in her case studies and examples. Using personable, jargon-free language that is easy to follow, she progressively explains the concepts of the Alexander Technique and their value in our busy world. Her book is a pleasure to read."

**Dr Terry Fitzgerald**

# Dedication

To my children Alison and Christopher,
and my sisters Brenda and Claire.

# Contents

# Acknowledgements

I thank many people who helped along the way with advice, opinions, suggestions and contributions. Everyone was very generous with their time, their willingness to be models for the photos and to try out some of my more crazy ideas to see what worked and what didn't. Thanks to them the ideas that didn't make sense are back in the brain grinder and may appear one day on a blog. Thanks to teachers and students of the Brighton Alexander Technique College. They include Astrid Holm for her creative writing and posture contribution and many helpful conversations about the Alexander Technique and posture, and for convincingly startling Francesca with a balloon and a needle!; Richard Boland for taking his shirt off so I could photograph his back whilst he played his violin – he assured me he had a wax especially for the photos; Francesca Aldridge for her article on eyesight and being a great model; and Rupert Ritchie, Janet Jacobs and Sherry Loh for modeling for me.

Thanks too to students Dai Richards, for modeling and sharing his thoughts on slacklines, unicycles and balance; Magdalena Elvinnson for showing us how to organize a long neck and back; Lola Lendinez for her modeling and remarkable story of recovery from a fractured neck, and giving us all hope that pain can be a thing of the past; and Trevelyan Harper keep a very good diary of his postural adventures, which happily turned out well for him. I'm grateful for his insights. Thanks to friend and colleague Stephanie Smith for her thoughtful contribution on posture and why it doesn't pay to be a slouch potato; pupils Marie and Rose for sharing their respective stories of horsemanship and professional violin playing – you can see clips of Marie on her marvellous horse Gabriel on YouTube. Grateful thanks to Matthew Andrews for his fantastic, insightful photos, which showed just what I wanted. It's easy to see which photos are his; they are the classically simple ones, lit beautifully on a white background. Finally, thanks to my children Christopher and Alison who have patiently endured postural experiments and conversations over the last year.

# Introduction

When I was asked to write another book about good body use, based on the Alexander Technique, I thought a great deal about what I wanted to say and how I wanted to say it. The word that kept popping into my head was 'posture'. People are very concerned about posture these days, and rightly so, but there is little of genuine help available to the intelligent student. Posture is a very subtle business and goes well beyond ideas of standing or sitting straight. Posture underpins everything you do – all your activities, such as swimming, horse riding, playing sport or music, as well as things you might not consider activities, such as breathing, circulation and digestion. It plays a part in back pain and other neuromuscular problems. For you to do anything at all you have to move; you have to use your body and your mind. You can't avoid it and you can't separate the two out.

In this book I aim to examine subtle postural tools and offer you ways you can use them in your own life. Over the years I have been teaching good use of the body, I have evolved a series of exercises that help people improve their awareness of what they are doing. This is often the first step to improving posture – an understanding that you might be holding tension in habit patterns that are so deeply ingrained in you they feel normal and you might not even believe you have them. So here, for the first time, I am offering these exercises to you. I hope they will become your manual for movement.

Carolyn Nicholls
Brighton
July 2012

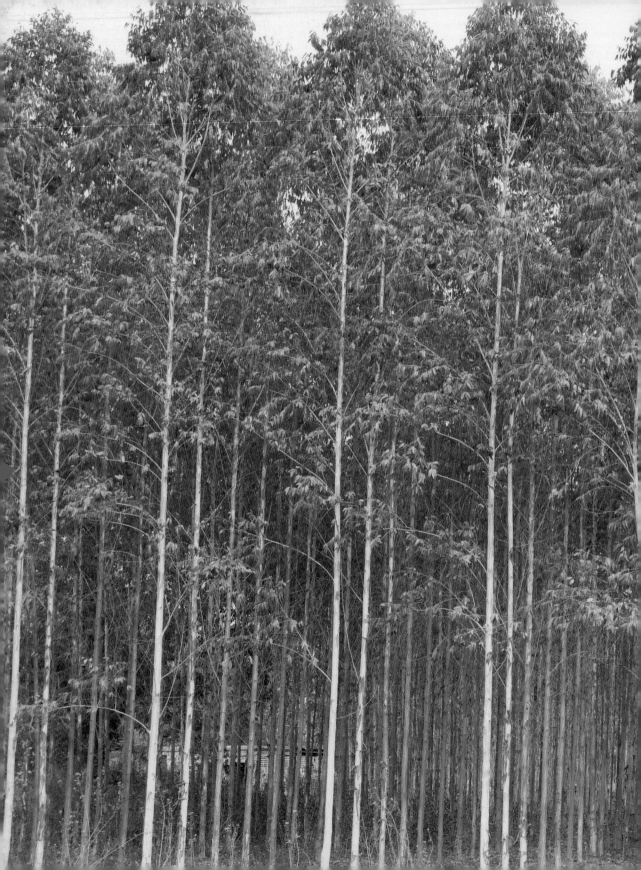

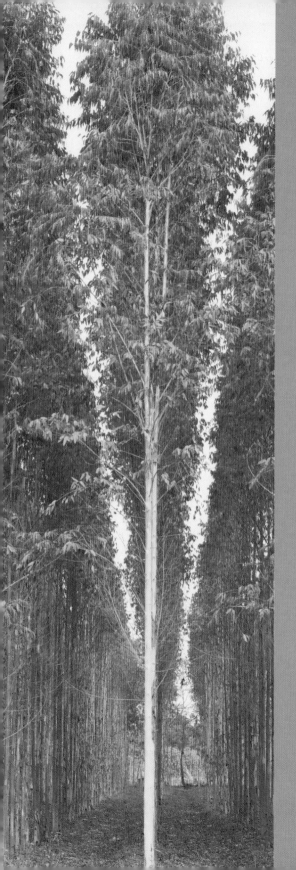

# Section 1

# Understand your posture

# Chapter 1
## Redefining posture

**This chapter covers:**
- what posture is
- the elements of our structure
- habits of mind and body
- how to improve posture through thought–posture–movement

## In search of better posture

Posture and body language are the first thing people notice about us. Confident people use their bodies differently from those who are diffident. A lack of confidence makes us shrink physically into ourselves. Our shoulders narrow, our neck droops forward on our shoulders and our head is retracted down onto our neck. This gives us a defeated look and people are less likely to listen to us if we project that bodily message. Most people are self-conscious about their posture. Either they believe their posture to be poor, or someone has told them it is. Very often people apologize for their posture or talk about it as if it were separate from them. 'Oh, I have terrible posture' is a common cry.

Posture is not a simplistic matter and the solutions to bad posture are not simple. They require thought. Poor posture deservedly gets a very bad press; back pain and other aches and pains are blamed on it. For many people, posture is the reason they seek out an Alexander teacher's help (see section 2). But what is posture? Is it about standing up straight, like soldiers on parade? Or pulling your shoulders back so they aren't rounded? Well, it's about more than that. It's a complex mixture of your individual structure, your habits of mind and body, your movement patterns, your breathing and all sorts of complex activities of your nervous system.

## Thought–posture–movement

Many things influence your posture. First there is your own structure, which is largely inherited, but accidents, illnesses, emotions and moods all play a part in creating your posture and are reflected in it. You will usually know if a friend is feeling unwell because they seem to shrink a little; their head and neck are withdrawn into hunched shoulders, and their whole body is slightly droopy. Their body tells you all you want to know about how they are. Posture says so much about us that actors put on and take off postures like a second skin to create their character. Who ever saw a super hero slouching? Not likely – they hold their head up, their chest is open and their shoulders broad. There is no twist or distortion in their back; they certainly don't stand leaning on one hip before they fly off to rescue the world. An actor portraying an unhappy character registers the emotions in their bodies – the bowed head, the hollow chest, the strained face. We all recognize what his body is telling us before he opens his mouth. Why? Because posture tells the world our story.

Most efforts at improving posture – for whatever reason – are either ineffective or short lived. This is mostly because we are often out of touch with exactly what we are doing with ourselves. Attempts to improve posture are made by changing the outside structure, and this always causes trouble. Our habits have such a strong grip on us that the subtleties of our head balance – a very important issue in posture – can pass us by. Our sensitivity can be so off kilter we simply don't know what we are doing. If we are holding ourselves up with excessive tension, this becomes almost hard wired into us, and it feels right and normal and any attempt to change it feels strange and wrong. If we approach things head on – for example by standing up straight or pulling our rounded shoulders back – we are unlikely to succeed because we are still doing the wrong things in the first place. We still have our old posture patterns and our tensions. We usually end up adding another layer of tension on the top of the one we already have, so we try harder and the trying gets us into even deeper trouble.

We need to find a more subtle way of going about things, an indirect way rather than a direct way, so we are changing things from the inside rather than the outside. To do this we have to recognize that posture is a matter not of external shape but of internal organization and this starts with our thinking. Understanding how to project messages to your muscles by directed thought is what informs posture, and posture is the lynch pin of movement. If we want to move well, either to walk about during our day or to do complex things like play instruments, or engage in demanding sports or exercise, our posture is a primary consideration. We will explore this process – thought–posture–movement – throughout this book. My thinking about posture has grown out of my understanding of the Alexander Technique. As a teacher and a trainer I have been involved in good body use for over 30 years.

# Postural role models

We learn posture largely unconsciously, through what we do on our journey from babyhood to upright walking toddler, child, young adult and fully grown individual. On the way to adulthood we model ourselves on our peer group and those whom we admire. If you have a slouching family this is what you see, accept and copy. Going out into the world as a young person your desire to fit in to your surroundings will encourage you to adopt the posture, body habits and body language of those around you whom you either admire or want not to offend. If you are in a situation where walking upright is not considered cool, then you won't walk upright. Many young people don't want to stand out from the crowd and so do whatever it takes to fit in, even if that includes doing uncomfortable things with their bodies, like slouching. Sadly, the consequences can outlast your peer group and long after the need to slouch in order to fit in has passed, you are still slouching. It's become a habit and one that is very hard to challenge and change.

The most usual motivation for changing posture is pain. Ultimately slouching will cause some sort of pain in most people. The long-term effects of compressing your body by slouching will be felt at some point. This can come as a surprise because habits are hard to recognize; it is difficult to believe they are damaging, but they are. It just takes time for them to catch up with you. You might get away with slouching your way through your 20s and develop back pain, or shoulder or neck pain, in your 30s. It can seem to you the pain comes out of the blue – but it didn't, it just got to the point where your unconscious misuse of your posture caught up with you.

# Posture of the past

Less than 100 years ago, an upright posture was considered normal; slouching just didn't happen.

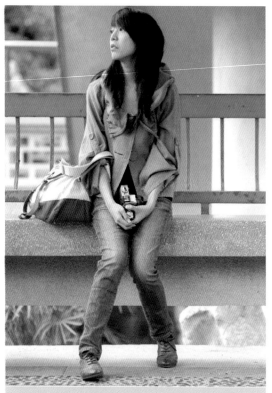

*The fashionable slouch may look cool, but with her head dragging down onto her neck, her shoulders drooped forward and her back compressed as a result, this woman's joints and internal organs will suffer.*

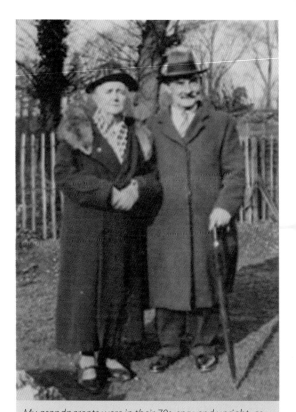

*My grandparents were in their 70s, spry and upright, as they had been all their lives. Both retain a long neck with their heads neither jutting forward nor dragged back, but held centrally. Their shoulders are wide and open, not hunched. They stand easily, with their feet taking their weight evenly. There are no twists or distortions in their frames. After a lifetime of physical labour, both retain freedom of movement in old age. They did not consider themselves unusual, or strive in any way to maintain their posture. An upright frame was their habit, and the habits of those around them. It is not the case now. The chairs they sat in all their lives were flat bottomed with upright backs. They sat very little, usually only to eat their meals; the rest of the time they would be moving around, although in the evenings they would sit in their upright Victorian chairs, my grandmother knitting and my grandfather reading. When they were schoolchildren they sat at desks with a slope to write on. They walked a great deal..*

Concepts of good posture are reflected in our language: 'a fine upstanding man' and 'a pillar of the community' are old fashioned phrases that reflect this. There was no question about it, you held yourself upright because everyone else did the same. From childhood to old age, your spine was straight.

# Posture is important

Posture has a profound effect on our health and wellbeing, but most people worry about the look of their posture and don't understand its far reaching implications. Poor posture contributes to back pain and other ills. It also influences

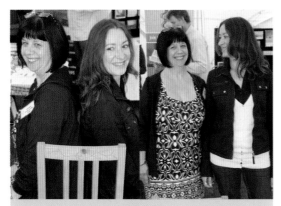

When Janet and Lola sit back to back, Janet is 'taller' because she has a long back. When they stand up, Lola's head and shoulders are higher than Janet's.

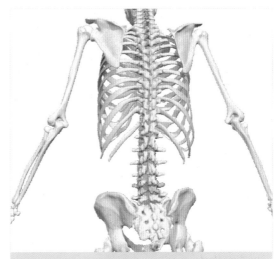

The fifth lumber vertebra is shown in pink. Notice how long the lumbar area is between the ribs and the pelvis. An extra vertebra here could make you even longer.

your breathing, digestion and circulation. Your posture directly affects the way you walk, run, play your instrument or sit at your computer.

Posture is more subtle than simply standing or sitting straight. It's the basis of all movement and activities. The impact of posture on your breathing is particularly important. As you age, you tend to use less of your lung capacity, which has a detrimental effect on many body systems. Most obvious are the oxygen levels in your blood. If your breathing is habitually shallow your whole system is sluggish. If you sit in a stuffy room, you generally feel sleepy and a bit stupid; you also feel tired and can't wait to get out, stretch and take in some real air. Shallow breathing is like putting your body in a stuffy room all the time. Your energy levels drop, and you can get into a depressive cycle where you lack energy because you don't have enough oxygen in your system, and so your lungs don't expel the waste products of your blood back into the air as efficiently as they should. That then makes you more sluggish and less inclined to move, which is the very thing you should be doing.

Movement and posture go hand in hand. Breathing and posture go hand in hand, too; it's a love triangle of the best kind. To be well, healthy and functioning easily, you need good posture,

good breathing and to move. Your body is made to move, not to spend all day in a chair.

This book presents for the first time detailed procedures used to change body use and posture profoundly. It explores aspects of posture in a practical way, rather than a theoretical one. It always helps to know a little bit about how we are made, how joints are designed to move and muscles to work, so we explore that too. It helps even more to know a bit about what they are not designed to do.

## Your structure

My sister was six foot tall, and she married a man who was five feet nine inches. When they sat side by side on their garden wall he was taller than her. But when they stood up, she was three inches taller than him. Her height was all in her long legs, a family feature, which has come down through the generations; 'Ah, yes, the Cannon legs,' we exclaim as the latest toddler in the family unfolds long limbs. He had a long back and short legs, and had all his trousers shortened. They were known as Miss Long Shanks and Mr Short **** (you have to guess that bit). Their individual structure made for different challenges in their lives, as will yours. This individuality is why so many chairs feel uncomfortable. Ironically, chairs that are often referred to as ergonomic are designed for the average person. I have yet to meet this person. If you sit in a chair designed to support your back, but your back isn't where the chair has decided it should be, then the chair won't feel comfortable and won't help your posture. Few of us can afford to have a chair tailor made for us – and even if we could, the moment we moved in it everything would change. So we have to be more intelligent about our posture in the world.

Everybody's structure is unique, as different from another person's as fingerprints. This is one reason why general advice on posture can be so unhelpful for some people and why we don't fit into ergonomic chairs. It would be nice to think we were all made the same way, and to a large extent we are. We all have a spine, with a head balancing on one end, a ribcage, shoulder and pelvic girdles and limbs; but our individual quirks and idiosyncrasies become our challenges, and we need intelligent ways of coping with them.

Just consider the number of lumber vertebrae you are supposed to have – most people have five, but some have six. Most of us have twelve pairs of ribs, but occasionally people have thirteen pairs. These variations might cause problems, or they might not, but if you have such a variation, you have to balance it out in your movement one way or another. Why do some people have longer backs than others, but are still short overall? It's more likely that each vertebra body is slightly longer than 'normal' than that they have an extra vertebra – but only an x-ray will tell that. Whether you do or don't have an extra vertebra, you still have to use it well.

## Long back, long neck

If you have a long back and a long neck you have to coordinate them well if you want to move easily without pain. If you are also lightly built you have more problems. Add on the possibility of lax ligaments and you are almost bound to run into problems. The word 'gangly' describes this structure nicely. Often it is used in relation to a teenager who has had a big growth spurt, which in itself can be the cause of back pain. For young women who shoot above their friends and above all the boys when they are teenagers, there is the added pressure of not wanting to be tall and consequently stooping, either intentionally or as a byproduct of shyness. Whatever the reason for this type of posture being adopted, it soon becomes fixed and hard to change. It can lead to scoliosis, where the spine curves unnaturally to the side, causing pain and problems. If people with scoliosis have distorted posture it creates harmful pressures on internal organs. Scoliosis can cause the ribcage literally to crush the lungs and put significant strain on the heart. If scoliosis is severe, surgery may be the only option.

## Case Study
### Kim's Story: when posture really counts

Most people are conscious of their posture, whether as a matter of appearance or because it contributes to back pain or digestive problems. Posture can be a serious health issue for a small number of people, although many have a small degree of scoliosis without any problems.

Kim was diagnosed with severe scoliosis when she was 15. The twist of scoliosis distorted her whole torso; her right shoulder was two inches in front of her left and tugged down into her waist. Her pelvis was twisted so when she stood, thinking she had her feet side by side, she didn't: one foot was in front of the other, and she suffered hip pain as a result of the uneven load on her leg joints.

Teenage scoliosis is measured in degrees. An x-ray of the spine is taken and the angle of 'tilt' is

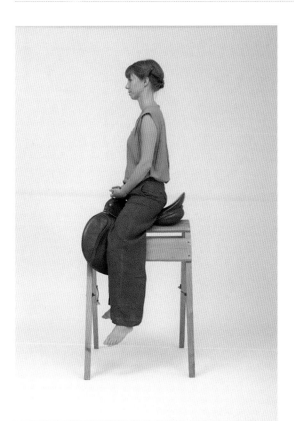

*A long back and long neck need good organization, as shown here. Mimi's head is poised on her long neck, which in turn is well balanced on the rest of her spine, right down to her sitting bones resting on the saddle. Her shoulder girdle is supported by her well-sprung spine so her arms don't drag on her neck. Her sitting bones and pelvis offer good support for her legs so they are able to lie freely on the saddle. If she were badly organized throughout her head, neck and back, sitting on the saddle would be uncomfortable.*

only did exercises, but had specialist lessons in the Alexander Technique. These two things worked together for her. Exercises can be very helpful if performed well, but if you are holding on to tension in different areas of your body because your posture is bad, exercises can actually make things worse. Kim learnt how to let her ribs move flexibly when she breathed, and how to maintain a good tone through her back muscles so she used her body in a coordinated way. This is slow work, but it can pay dividends. The last time Kim was measured, the distortion was 28 degrees. This was very good news, but Kim still had to work at her postural support continuously. Like many teenage girls with scoliosis, Kim is tall, nearly six foot, very slender and she has somewhat lax ligaments, and a growth spurt! The Alexander lessons can help her manage all that in a positive way, and can be applied to her exercises and movement when she is walking, or sitting to study. Posture is always with you, no matter what you are doing. Kim still needs monitoring by her orthopaedic specialist and she wears the corset specially designed for her. She is very fit and active and has little pain. The important thing for her is to move in a coordinated way, otherwise her activity will make her distortion worse by reinforcing the 'muscle memory' her body holds.

Kim continued with her lessons for a full year and then it became obvious she did need surgery. She was not disappointed as she felt she had such a lot she could do to help herself, and the year of learning also gave her time to accept her situation. Kim had no pain, apart from in her hip, which was resolved quickly, so it wasn't easy for her to see the need for surgery.

Each case is very different. After her surgery Kim was keener than ever to apply her Alexander knowledge to her posture and activities and she recovered so quickly her surgeon was impressed.

calculated. Anything over 48 degrees deviation from normal (0 degrees) is serious enough for surgery to be considered. Kim's spine was 44 degrees, a significant problem. The distorted torso can press on internal organs, restricting the heart and lungs, which can be affected by the increased internal pressure. For girls, this could significantly threaten future pregnancies.

Seeking skilled help with her posture, Kim not

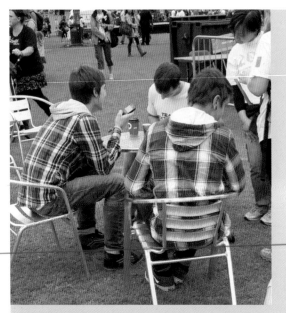

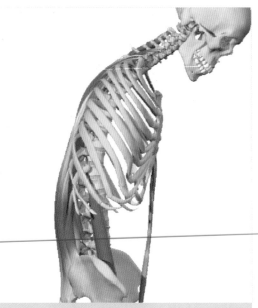

*Sitting like this might seem comfortable when you are young, but you are putting unnecessary and excessive pressure on your neck and lower back. One day it will*

*complain. Look what is happening to the skeletal system when you sit in a heap. What is being squashed internally is even more significant.*

These are some facts about scoliosis:

- Most scoliosis is not painful and is only picked up in examinations, perhaps by a school nurse.
- Scoliosis can be hereditary. If it's in your family – watch out for it!
- Good management is the key to coping.
- Don't ignore it – you will not grow out of it and it will not go away without skilled help

# Habits of mind and body

Some humans love routines; others hate them and seek to avoid them. Our posture and the way we move are largely dominated by our routine ways of doing things, our habits of mind and body. Did you know you can practice tension? If you habitually clench all your muscles, after a while

you don't notice it – but you carry on practicing tension until you are really good at it – and then trouble begins. Winding your legs round the legs of your chair when you sit down is a habit, but not a useful one. The first few times you do it you won't notice anything and it won't hurt you, but as a constant habit, it will put pressure on your back as you sit and re-enforce tension in your legs. This can reduce blood flow to your pelvic area, which is not a good thing. Crossing your legs is often so unconscious a habit it can be hard to break. There is no harm in crossing your legs for a short time if you want to – but if you feel more comfortable with your legs always crossed it's likely to be because your legs are very tense. If that is the case you are likely to want to cross your legs even if you know it's not a good idea. Familiar tension slips below our awareness radar and takes us straight back into our habits.

What if your habit is to pull your body down as you walk or stand? What does this mean to you and why is it a bad idea? This brings us back to

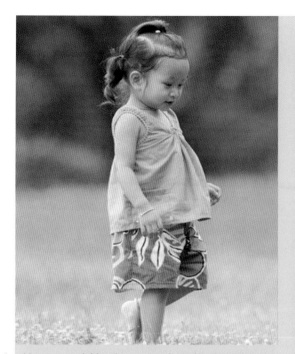

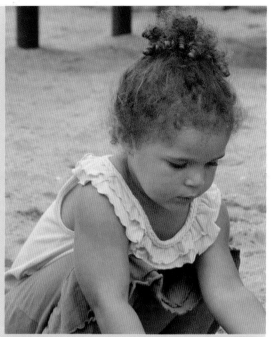

*Most young children have natural good body use, but with a lack of good role models and the prevalence of poor posture all around, it's not hard to see why things go wrong. Good head poise is natural to most youngsters: there is no stiffness in the top 'nodding joint' of the head; their backs are naturally straight; and joints bend easily to allow them to walk, run, squat and perform any movement without pain. Their attention is mostly on exploring their world in a way that is largely tactile, rather than listening to an adult. This natural good use stays with some people for far longer than others, and if you are fortunate to have an easy structure to cope with you may not suffer too much, but as children are introduced to the terrors of sitting still (not a natural thing for a young person), things can start to deteriorate very quickly.*

the effects of poor body use and posture on the things you can't see, such as your lungs, digestive system, circulation and joints. If you habitually stoop, or pull your lower back in with tension, the overall effect is to shorten you. This is easily seen from the outside. What is not visible at all is the extra compression on your joints, the consequent restriction of your respiratory system, and the squashing of your internal organs – which don't like it by the way. You will not notice what you are doing, it might not cause immediate problems, but you could be storing up trouble for later. By the time someone gets to the point of debilitating pain they have been carrying themselves around badly for a long time. If you have the tension habit,

you constantly practice it. Every time you practice it, it feels more natural and undoing it takes time and can be a strange experience.

A drooping neck encourages stiffness in the shoulders, and a depression of the upper thorax so breathing is subtly suppressed. Just this one fact has far reaching consequences. Over a period of time it leads to poor breathing patterns, which reduces lung capacity, makes ribs and diaphragm stiff and impedes free digestion. This drooped neck is sometimes referred to as 'text neck', and might be linked to overuse of texting and computer use generally. The drooped neck is an obvious sign of a pattern of misuse that runs through the whole body.

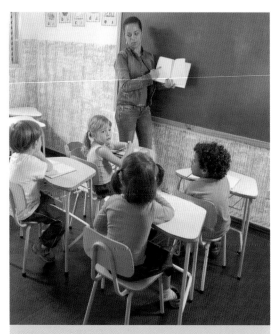

*These youngsters are already sitting badly with slouched backs and heads compressed down onto their necks. It is difficult to see the necks of any of the four children, as they are squashed down onto their shoulders. The chairs make it difficult for the children to get support from the floor because they are badly designed for the young bodies that occupy them. Their desks are too high for them so it's a strain to write or draw. Their elbows get pushed up into their shoulders by the desks – they can't be comfortable. Their role model teacher is slouching too – she's actually leaning on the blackboard to hold herself up! What kind of message does that give? It doesn't have to be like that.*

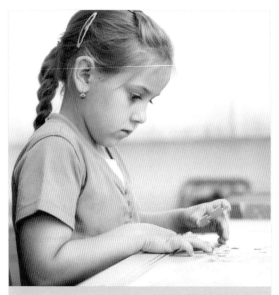

*This young girl is sitting upright easily, with her back supporting her and her head angled easily so she can see her jigsaw pieces. Her hands and arms are used naturally because the chair is the correct height for her body, so she has space for her back to lengthen naturally. She can easily keep her neck long, even though she won't be thinking about it.*

## Your body wants to balance

However you hold yourself, your body will seek a balance. If you constantly drop your neck forward, your shoulders will hunch up to give some support, your neck muscles will tighten up to support the weight of your head and your whole torso will distort underneath your head and neck to compensate for what is going on in your body. Are you achieving your balance in an easy way that lets you move pain free and easily, or are you compensating for one problem by creating a whole load of others? And has this compensation become such a habit you no longer notice it? If it has you have jumped on to the bad habit merry-go-round where you do the things you do with your body because that's what you have done for such a long time it feels right.

# The bad habit merry-go-round

## The unconscious tension habit...

If you are habitually over-tense, you have successfully taught yourself that excessive tension is normal. It is interesting to consider just how much tension is normal and how you are

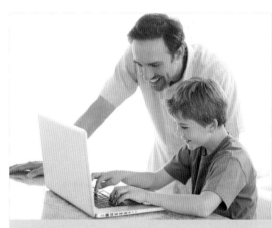
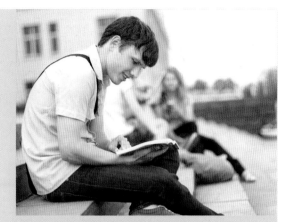

If you have started slouching when very young, you are unlikely to stop, most likely because you are unaware of it and those around you are oblivious of it too. The young boy sitting at his dad's computer may look happy but already his shoulders are rounded, his neck is dropped forward and his upper back is as rounded as his dad's. A few years of this and he will be sitting in a big C curve, like the lad reading on the steps. It doesn't take a postural genius to spot that this isn't healthy. Postural habits like these are quickly formed and because they are constantly practiced are very hard to change, especially as so many people have no idea what causes them, or what they might do about them. Both these young boys already show signs of the most common postural distortion, where the column of the neck is drooped forward on the shoulders.

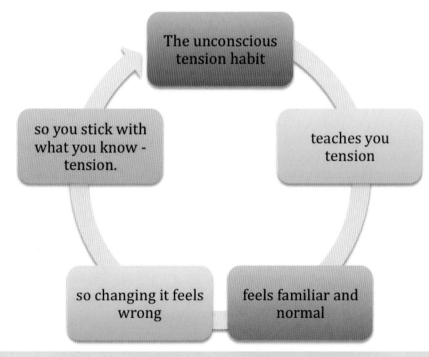

*The bad habit merry-go-round*

applying it to yourself. Let's consider a balance between appropriate tone, or muscular effort and inappropriate tension. The route of poor posture is often excessive tension in everyday activities that don't need it, such as simply walking quietly, or even lying in bed. It is possible to do these things with a damaging degree of tension, simply because you have taught yourself that tension is normal. Every time you do something, like walking, lying in bed or maybe lolling around on the sofa, you practice excessive tension, because that is what you have been doing for some time. Its familiarity can even feel comforting: 'It's the way I am', you might say to yourself.

## ...teaches you tension...

Our nervous system constantly learns from what we do. It would be nice to think it only learned the good things, but this is not the case. Habit can be a friend or a monster. If you consistently walk with your neck stiff and your head retracted, you reinforce the message to yourself that this is the best way to walk – just like the habitual smoker lighting up without even realizing it, you don't notice it. Sadly, you can't throw your neck tension and bad habits in the bin – but there are things you can do! If you play a favorite sport, such as golf or tennis, with postural tension, you will find giving up your tension a real challenge. You may even convince yourself you need it in order to play. You don't. What you need is well coordinated, fluid, functioning muscles throughout your body, operating at the right tone level for your activity. Not tension!

## ...which feels familiar and normal...

This is where our sensory awareness can deceive us and ultimately we have to challenge sensory awareness if we want to break our tension habit. When something feels familiar and normal it also feels right, and to a certain degree emotionally comforting. If you have developed the habit of

walking around with your neck dropped forward you may be startled to see a sideways-on photo of yourself, which reveals just how bad the droop is. When they are unknowingly photographed in side profile many people are shocked by what they see and say, 'I thought I was standing up straight.' It takes time to challenge deeply ingrained habits.

## ...so changing it feels wrong...

A corollary of the familiar sensations we have from our habitual posture is the sensation that anything different we attempt feels wrong. This encourages us to go back to the previous habit, just because it is familiar and our senses tell us it's 'right', even though we know its 'wrong'. When you think about changing your posture and body use, you may have to experience a period of time where you feel the new changes are definitely wrong. It doesn't mean they are wrong.

## ...so you stick with what you know – tension

It's always easier to do what you know. But when you have based that 'knowing' on faulty sensory awareness it's not useful to keep doing it. First you have to understand what it is you are likely to be doing, regardless of what you feel you are doing, and then you have to set up thought pathways leading to actions that help you change what you are doing. You will need to delve deeper into your habits than you might have thought.

## You don't need to stay that way

Your brain loves learning, and as a species we are endlessly adaptable. This can work for us if we understand it. If you have held yourself badly for years, you will have built up a lot of what you could call holding patterns. You have taught yourself to be this way. You can also teach yourself not to stay that way. Even small shifts in awareness can offer a new insight into how you move and hold yourself. In essence, we are adaptable and

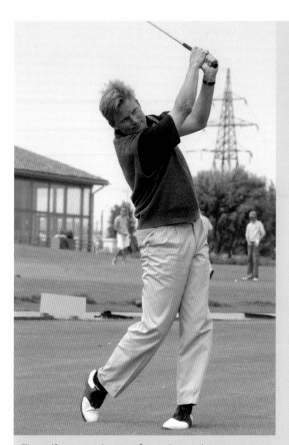
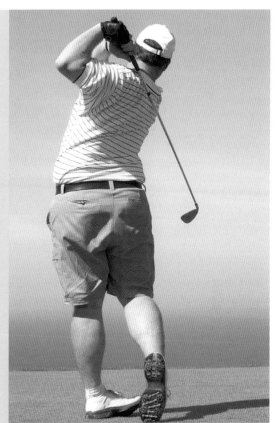

The golf swing makes significant demands on your body. It can create pressure in the hip of your supporting leg, strain on both knees, tightness across the shoulders and a damaging compressive twist in your back. As always, it's not what you do, but how you do it. To put it another way, the things you are already doing with yourself – which you might call your posture or your use – will profoundly influence not only the success of your golf swing but also what it does to you. The golfer on the left has an easy flow of upright movement through his structure and demonstrates nicely that good posture is not a matter of standing in a straight line. Despite the demands of the golf swing, which twists the body in several ways, he nevertheless has good coordination between his head, neck and back; they are working in harmony with each other.

The golfer on the right shows the opposite. His whole direction of muscular energy is downwards, not upwards. This has resulted in the twist in his back being full of tension and effort. In the long run, this will cause him problems. A clue to his tension is also seen in his supporting foot, the toes of which are off the ground. When he runs into back problems, he may well think that the golf has caused them. But it hasn't – the cause is the way he uses his body – which he does not change whether he's playing golf or not. If he wants to avoid back pain when playing, he has to address the underlying issues.

the idea that you can't teach an old dog new tricks has been proved wrong over and over again. All it takes is a bit of willingness on your part to try something different – to experience a new way of moving, so that instead of surrendering to habitual tension, you challenge it in yourself.

F. M. Alexander, after whom the Alexander Technique is named, was a postural genius, and his gift to us is that he worked out what habitual tension does to the human being. His insights were, and still are, profound. His findings pointed the way to how anyone who is willing to be thoughtful about it can unravel the tangle of postural difficulties for themselves. I have taught people in their 80s as well as people aged under 10, and once they become aware of what they are unintentionally doing to themselves, which either contributes to or totally creates their difficulties, they are on a new path, which leads to change. Habits form quickly, particularly in relation to a chosen activity, such as guitar playing. Your everyday habits will determine how you play, and how you play will then affect your everyday habits. So if you slump over your guitar and hold your wrist stiffly, you are likely to continue to slump and hold your wrist stiffly when you eat your dinner or do the washing up. This stiffness will feel normal, so you'll carry on with it – maybe to the point of pain or injury.

## Case Study
### Brian learned confidence

Posture and body language are the first thing people notice about us. Confident people use their bodies differently from those who are diffident. Lack of confidence makes us shrink physically into ourselves. This gives us a defeated look and people are less likely to listen to us if we project that bodily message. When Brian sought help, he hoped improving his body use would help his confidence, and went on to say he knew

he had terrible posture and his girlfriend thought it made him look shy.

On meeting Brian, I could see what his girlfriend meant – he was tall and slender and very collapsed; his upper back was rounded and his lower back pulled in. It made him look a lot older than he was. He had a very slight scoliosis. He'd had an enormous growth spurt as a teenager and became very lanky and uncoordinated, and had back and leg pain. His mates nicknamed him spider because of his long arms and legs, which he hated. Now in his early 30s he still had mild back pain and a lanky look.

Teaching Brian to support his back and neck differently was a challenge. He was so used to the way he carried himself that all his efforts to move differently felt wrong and occasionally painful. He persisted, was diligent with his active rest practice (one of your postural five-a-day, described in Chapter 10) and came in for his tenth lesson with a huge smile on his face saying his back felt completely different. He had both lengthened and widened, and his shoulders had opened out. He looked much more relaxed and confident. He said he had some posture tools to help him in difficult situations, whenever he felt tense or nervous. Instead of shrinking into himself – which was his old response – he released the tension in his neck muscles, reminded himself to 'think up', checked out what he was doing with his feet and made sure he wasn't holding his breath.

Brian's awareness of his body use continued to improve as he had more lessons. He took up the guitar again, something he'd enjoyed but stopped because it gave him back pain. He was more outgoing, confident and willing to try new things. He had started lessons because of back pain and lack of confidence, and now he applied his new knowledge to all sorts of aspects of his life, including a career change. He decided to give up being a banker and instead to train to be a body therapist. As he commented, you never know what doors open when you start changing.

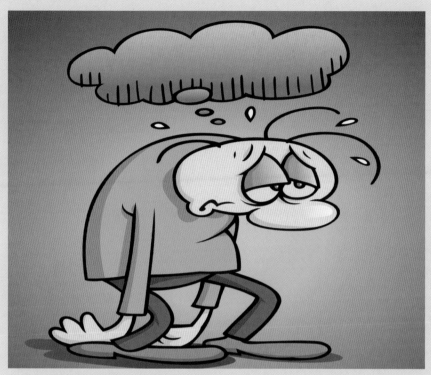

*Even cartoon people reveal their mental and emotional state through their posture.*

# Pathways to better posture: thought–posture–movement

The four main elements that make up our posture are our structure, the way we use ourselves, our breathing and our habits. Life throws challenges at us in the form of accidents, stress and illness, all of which have an effect on our posture. Although you can't avoid these things you can help yourself to minimize them having a negative impact on your health. If you have a very long back and neck, or you have had an accident of some sort, you still have the basic facts of your coordination and movement to contend with. Putting thought and awareness into your postural habits will go a long way to improve your wellbeing, lift your spirits and allow you to do what you want in a pain free way. Posture is a matter of well-being – that elusive feeling you recognize when life is easy, you enjoy your challenges and cope with them. Our chosen posture is exactly that – chosen. You need to understand and apply the formula thought–posture–movement.

# Chapter 2
# Thought–posture–movement

The sequence thought–posture–movement can be used to describe the way we function and move ourselves around and to offer us a map to illuminate the territory. Put simply, movement comes about in response to an intention. For example, you want a cup of tea so you go into the kitchen and set about the tea-making task. You have probably done this so often you are on automatic pilot and don't really think about it. But to end up with your cup of tea a whole series of movements, adjustments and decisions take place. As you lift the empty kettle you judge very accurately how much effort you need – you won't lift it so forcefully that you throw it over your shoulder. Your nervous system is constantly relaying information from your body – for example about the weight of the kettle, which determines how far you should lift your hands – back to your brain. Your brain then sends back information to your body telling it how much muscular effort to use, what movements of joints are helpful and so on. It does this constantly, refining and changing the information from moment to moment. As you fill the kettle with water it gets heavier and you adjust to the extra weight without realizing you are doing so.

When you watch a young child encountering these challenges for the first time you can see how quickly and easily they learn. A young child on the beach soon learns that a bucket full of sea water

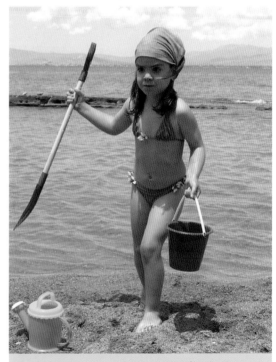

*This little girl is supporting the weight of her bucket by bending the elbow of her supporting arm. This enables her to keep the weight closer to her body and therefore makes it easier for her to carry the bucket. This is not a conscious act on her part; it comes about as practice shows her it's easier than having her arm straight. Even though you can't see inside the bucket you know it's full of water (or maybe sand) because you can see how she is using her body.*

is heavier than an empty bucket, and if they wish (intend!) to carry the water to their sandcastle, they will keep adjusting their hold on the bucket and their body stance until they can carry it without spilling a drop of their precious cargo. How do they do this?

# Chains of events

When you form an intention (making that cup of tea), it acts a stimulus. Stimuli come in all sorts of forms. They can come from within, for example your desire for tea, or from without, for example when someone asks you to make tea for them. They can be simple or complex. Heat and cold are stimuli and you will respond to them accordingly by taking off a layer of clothing or going to fetch another jumper. All living things respond to stimuli and we are no different – only more complex.

Let's say the stimulus has arisen in your mind and you are going to act on it. What happens? You have the thought, and to enact that thought your muscles and joints – your whole body – must move you to the kitchen, so your brain sets about sending an enormous amount of information to your muscles through your nervous system. It's a subtle and highly complex process involving all sorts of interactions, but much of it is information travelling back and forth along the physical pathways of your nervous system and brain. Your hands, feet, back – in fact all of you – are wired up for movement to take place as a result of your intentions.

# Learning pathways

Nerves convey messages from your brain to your muscles. If you have ever had a pinched nerve in your neck you'll know it affects not just your neck but your arm and hand too. They are two-way streets that convey information back to your brain about where you are in space and what you

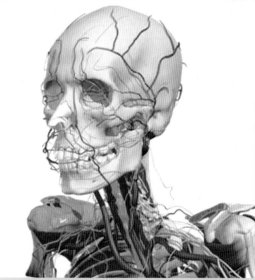

*This picture shows the tangle of nerves in cream, and arteries in red. Although this is a representational diagram you can see a huge number of nerves arising from the neck area, covering the face and feeding off down the arms on the way to the wrists, hands and fingers.*

are holding or touching. When your fingers and hands reach for the tea bag they are sensitive to its fragility compared with the teacup, so you adjust how much effort you use when handling the two different materials. This too is a learned skill. A child has to learn to stroke a puppy gently, but once she has done so she's unlikely to revert to rough handling.

The delicacy or firmness of touch is achieved by how much muscular effort you make, which is partly a matter of learning and partly a matter of consciousness. By the time you get to the age where you might lift a teacup you will have lifted many drinking vessels and have some sense of how heavy it's likely to be. When you lift it and take a sip, you have changed its weight, so when you put it down it's lighter than when you lifted it up. You will accommodate to that difference without even thinking about it because your nervous system has practiced this skill of adaptation and inhibition. Towards the end of the drink your cup is considerably lighter because it's almost empty, but you are unlikely to make errors in how much effort you use in your actions.

Inhibition is a refining skill of the nervous system that allows us to select the appropriate amount of effort for what we need to do. This is really a remarkable skill and transfers to all activities, not just tea drinking. You open doors with the right amount of effort. You carry shopping and still manage to walk up and down stairs without falling over. You pick things up, put them down, but your balance is rarely disturbed by your activities.

## Consciousness

Consciousness is not easily defined and this book is not intended to go deeply into the subject from a philosophical or neurophysiological perspective, but considers it as a practical tool that we can enhance. Most of the time we can choose how we respond to stimuli by making choices that suit us best. If we are cold we can go and get a jumper or have a hot drink to warm us up from the inside, or we choose to stay cold. This ability to choose is enhanced when we have time to make our decisions. Consciousness offers us an ability to respond to stimuli in a sophisticated way instead of thoughtlessly. We think of choice mostly as relating to external things – shall I have tea or coffee? – but it can apply to internal choices such as tension levels and muscle tone. Conscious awareness can help us to complete tasks with the minimum effort required.

## Inner world, outer expression

You really can't separate mind from body; there is no activity that uses only one or the other. Even if you think you are 'only thinking,' your facial muscles

are operating and your postural muscles are allowing you to sit in your chair. Likewise, although we yearn to 'switch off' occasionally, we never stop thinking – or rather our brain never stops being active. Our inner world of thoughts, feelings and emotions is reflected in our body, both in the way we hold ourselves, which you might call posture, and the way we move. It goes further than posture and movement; it also affects our functioning. If you are upset for any reason, you will find it affects you not only physically through tension but also functionally; you might lose your appetite or find your digestion has slowed down. Long-term mental tension creates long-term muscular tension, which in turn affects circulation, breathing and digestion. F. M. Alexander once said, 'You translate everything, whether physical, mental or spiritual, into muscular tension.'

Just as your nervous system is a two-way messenger between your brain and your body, and thoughts, emotions and habits reveal themselves physically, so you can use your body to influence your feeling and habits. If you are depressed, it will show in your drooped shoulders, shallow breathing and slack muscles. In other words, your posture will show what is going on in your mind. But if you find a way to change your posture, to lengthen your torso instead of compressing it, to open out your hunched shoulders, then it will affect your mood, and you will feel better. Just how you set about making those changes is the subject matter of this book.

## Body mapping

Body mapping is a way of exploring and discovering how your joints, muscles and tendons move in relation to each other. It is a useful skill, which can help you tune in to the function, mobility, injury and expression that is going on in your body. People have used the idea to help them tune into themselves in a variety of ways, for example by drawing around your outline when

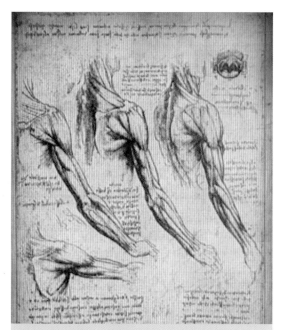

*This is a page from one of Leonardo da Vinci's sketchbooks. His study shows how muscles of the shoulder, neck and back respond to arm movement. It is a literal map of the body, and would have helped him make accurate paintings. Supposing Leonardo could paint you today, how would you look? What would your posture be like? When you get a shock catching sight of your profile in a shop window it could be because you are confronted with the mismatch in your body.*

lying on a huge sheet of paper and then writing or drawing about how you feel or where bits of you hurt and so on. The concept has been used to help assess injuries at work and indentify unsafe work practices. For example, a factory used body mapping to identify that their workers had a significant number of calf injuries. On investigation staff discovered that a particular shelf was stacked with sharp objects exactly at calf height. Until they had mapped out the injuries, no one had noticed this problem.

Artists draw the anatomy of the human figure to help them understand how people are put together and move. This is observation by the artist of another person from the outside. This doesn't mean the artist has a good understanding of their own body, but it is helpful for us to observe ourselves from the inside.

Body mapping can help you identify not only your relationship to the world around you, but also the relationships of parts within you.

Your thoughts and habits create a map of your body that you operate on to get around. Sometimes it isn't accurate; for example you underestimate the depth of a step and step down as if it were shallower than it really is – so you stumble – or you underestimate your height and crack your head passing through a low doorway. These mismatches between you and the world around you generally come out of a mismatch between you and you! By this I mean you may have little idea of where your joints are and this will affect how you use them and therefore how you move. Take hip joints; if you believe them to be higher up than they actually are – a common error – then you are likely to hold your real hip joints very stiffly while your body bends where it 'thinks' your hip joints are. This will affect the way you walk, sit, climb stairs or make any movement that involves your hip joints.

## Mapping your knuckles

You can body map your own hand to find out more about it. Are you sure you know how it bends? Hold your hand out in front of you with your fingers straight and your palm facing the floor. Look at the back of your hand. Flap your straight fingers down and up so they bend at the knuckle and notice where the joint is – it looks as if it's at the top of your hand, doesn't it?

Now turn your hand over so your palm faces upwards, with your fingers straight, and just look at it. Ask yourself where you think it will bend when you repeat that flapping action you just made. Unless you have done this before you are most likely to assume your fingers will bend at the point where they join your hand – right at the top of the palm.

Go ahead – bend your fingers – your hand bends

almost halfway down your palm! Not where you thought at all.

Most of the things we do with our hands give us a view of the back or side of them, so we might not fully realize where these joints are. Not knowing affects how we use our hands, especially if we are performing a sophisticated task such as playing an instrument. An unconscious assumption of where your knuckles bend can restrict your flexibility, so if you have stiff fingers from typing or playing the piano, look at this joint – is your map a little wrong? Could knowing where the joints really are help you move your hand and fingers with more ease? The answer is yes!

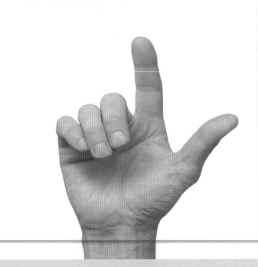

*Hand with three fingers bent forward and the first finger and thumb outstretched.*

## Occupational hazards

When you engage in an activity repeatedly and use your body poorly because your sense of it is not accurate, your map gets more and more distorted. This is particularly true of your head and neck. If you bring your head down to your camera when you take photographs and you do it by pulling your neck column forward, as the photographer in the shot opposite is demonstrating, this is your 'map' not only for taking photos but also for bringing things up to your face – mobile phones, headphones, knives and forks! Your map tells you to pull your neck forward, but your map is wrong!

## Why do we get stuck?

Given that we have such a flexible and adaptable communication between body and mind it is not easy to see why we run into such problems with our posture and breathing, but obviously we do. One of the reasons is that our flexible nature is essentially a learning nature and we constantly reinforce – or teach – ourselves ways to do things, for example supporting our bodies against the ever-present force of gravity. If we unwittingly teach ourselves

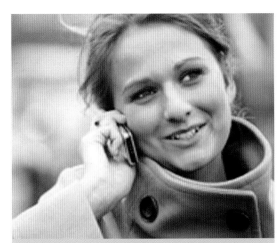

*Seeing people chatting on their mobile phone is so common you hardly notice it, and some people spend a considerable time each day doing exactly that. In this photograph, the woman is holding her head down on one side, pulling it down towards the phone. It may be because she has a mismatch about what her neck is doing so she fails to realize how distorted it is – or she may not understand that her shoulder has much more freedom than she is using and if she lifted it a bit more she could rise her arm up to her head easily.*

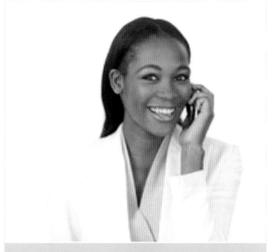

This woman's neck is not distorted and she has used her shoulder joint to bring her hand right up to her ear.

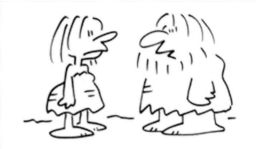

"IT WAS A VERY DEPRESSING CLASS REUNION -- I WAS THE ONLY ONE THERE WALKING UPRIGHT!"

Reflection on a class reunion.

that slumping is a good way to carry ourselves, then that's what we learn. It is very unlikely that you intend to slump, but if you have got into that habit the biggest problem you face is that slumping feels natural to you. It feels correct and any attempt you make to change it feels wrong.

This can be a difficult phase to get past because you need new awareness tools to cope with it. As creatures of habit we are also rather lazy and prefer to do what we know than something we don't. To make changes in our posture we must tackle our awareness and mental habits, and cultivate new ways of thinking. You may think these things don't matter but they do – over a period of time, a mismatch in your awareness leads to problems that really show in your posture.

# Practice a new way of thinking

Building a new way of thinking is largely a matter of practice – like any skill. It helps if you make a regular routine. The best way to learn this new way of thinking is in simple activities such as active rest, which is explained in detail in the second section of this book. The reason active rest works so well is that it is undemanding and so you can give your attention to your new thought process. But you

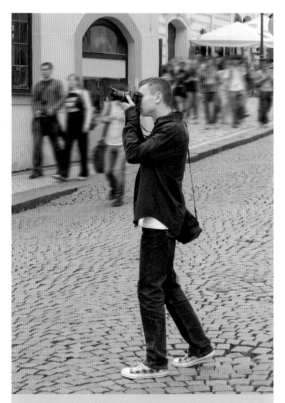

Dragging your head and neck towards the camera distorts your delicate head/neck/back relationship and can cause neck or back pain.

can experiment in any situation.

What you are really wanting is to do things – anything – with less tension and more direction. If you are casually walking down the street you could give some thought to your overall stature. Ask yourself if you are pulling your body down towards the ground. This is often unintentional and you may not notice it. If you never question yourself, you certainly won't notice, but even posing the question to yourself at a mental level increases your awareness. So next time you are walking see if you can ask yourself to walk tall, rather than slump. At first this will seem effortful and you won't have much way of telling if you are successful or not, but small amounts of time thinking in this way will build up new habits and lead to postural change. Your self-exploration becomes your self re-education.

# What kind of thought?

We use our minds in many different ways: we can concentrate, daydream, think of one thing while doing something completely different, focus sharply on a task or do it as we say 'half-heartedly'. This flexibility is part of our neurophysiology and plasticity and one of the things that make us live and express ourselves with such diversity, and it enables us to create our individuality. Our capacity to think in a variety of ways and the fact that we express our thoughts physically in our bodies is at the root of the formula thought–posture–movement. Our thoughts link to our emotions and we react to both. Our reactions always take place in our bodies, even if we don't immediately notice them; as soon as we tune into ourselves we experience this deep connection.

Think about something that makes you angry – or just think about the word 'angry' and notice what it does to you; you are likely to find your jaw tensed, your back muscles clenched and your breath held. Now think of a warm summer day, and you will feel different; your jaw will relax, you

might even smile. Your muscles will be less tense and you will notice a different kind of mood.

Understanding this link allows you to choose the manner of thinking that is most helpful. We are highly creative beings (even if we don't believe it!) and when we use our thinking in a focused way we can do a lot to help our posture and therefore our movement. So how can we harness this talent to our best advantage?

# Experiment in thinking

The kind of thinking that helps most is directed thinking, which is a skill involving awareness as well as projecting specific thoughts. This is different from visualization or simple observation. You can for example think about your wrist. Try it, just think about your wrist. Don't think anything in particular. The most likely result you will get is that your mind is drawn to your wrist and you become more aware of it; you might notice it tingling or feeling warm in response to your thinking about it. This kind of thinking improves your awareness and can make you more sensitive to tension and fatigue, but you can do more. Your clever brain has endless possibilities to explore.

Now try something a little different. Instead of just thinking about your wrist, give your wrist some direction that you 'send' from your mind. Ask your wrist to 'open' so that it decompresses and there is more space in it, so your hand is also more free to move. This kind of thinking takes practice but will give a very different result. Instead of awareness on its own – which is a good first step, and can take you a long way – you can refine this mind–body connection so you have the ability to influence your wrist in the way you choose. You could decide to tighten it up! I don't recommend that but you might choose to do so.

This way of thinking is not the same as visualization, where you might use an image to enhance your experience – for example visualizing your wrist being flexible and warm. This may be a useful skill but it isn't the same as directing your wrist to release. With directed thinking you are using your nervous system's wiring in the way it already exists. In other words, the pathways (between brain and wrist in this case) are already there and you are bringing those pathways into focus more clearly. As you do this, you also strengthen the pathways, so the next time you ask your wrist to release, it does so more easily.

The implications of this link between mind and muscle are far reaching and offer us scope to influence our posture and functioning on a subtle level. The link also reminds us that if we do nothing with our minds, or are unaware of this powerful link, we are leaving our posture and function to chance and habit, and sadly that doesn't always serve us well.

## Finger-tip experiment

This is a simple but powerful experiment that demonstrates the way we can take advantage of the existing link between thinking in a directed, focused way, which sends a message from mind to muscle, and the response in our bodies.

You need a friend, an A4 sheet of paper, a pencil and a flat surface. To get the best result from this experiment you need to sit in balance, at a desk or table, on a flat-bottomed chair with your feet flat on the floor. Take a moment to 'find' your sitting bones at the base of your pelvis and balance over them, so you are sitting gently upright. You are not forcing anything but you are ensuring you are not slumping in a heap.

Sit down and place your flat palm on the sheet of paper with your fingers straight. Now ask your friend to draw a line with the pencil round your fingertips, as close as you can get. Then close your eyes. Make sure you don't hold your breath and don't deliberately move your hand!

Now 'direct' your wrist to 'open', just as you did in the previous experiment. Then 'direct' your fingers and thumb to lengthen away from your open wrist. Take a little time over this; it's not something you can rush. Most people will feel as if their hand

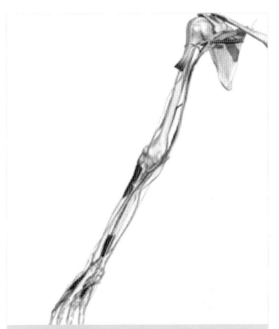

*In this diagram the nerve pathway from your neck to your wrist, hand and fingers is shown in cream and green. When you send a directed thought to your wrist, you use this pathway. When you 'link up' your thinking so the message is consciously sent from your mind down your arm to your wrist, you are not only using the existing pathway to your best advantage but also making it easier and easier to do so.*

is creeping up the paper a little. After a short time, ask your friend to draw round your fingertips again, and when she has finished, open your eyes and remove your hand.

Did it work for you? Most people get a measurable increase in the length of their fingers merely by 'asking' for it to happen. Your hand is a highly sensitive part of your body and you are likely to notice these changes. Now pick up the pencil and continue to ask your wrist to stay 'open' while you write your name on the paper. The experience of lengthening your hand should make it feel a little different when you write.

# Whole body thinking

This skill you have just discovered is the basis for your new postural awareness and improvement. Instead of thinking in 'bits', you learn what is the most important coordination to apply your thinking to – the crucial coordination of your head, neck and back. When you understand the structure you have to work with, and the best way to use it, you are well on your way to making significant changes in posture, breathing, circulation, digestion and, most importantly, reducing your likelihood of aches and pains and overuse injuries.

# Threading thought into movement

Most people think of movements as large acts – such as walking, dancing or picking something up. But even when you are sitting still you continue to move. Inside you your heart beats, your ribs move as you breathe, your digestive system works and muscles hold you up. The idea of becoming aware of thought as something useful to consider before you move helps influence your posture in a positive way. It doesn't mean you have to aspire to a level of super consciousness and not take a step without working out how to do it – that would be extremely tedious and robotic, and we are much cleverer than even the most advanced robots when it comes to movement (they are better at maths…). This pathway, thought – posture – movement, is what happens naturally and becoming more aware of it helps us.

You may wonder how your posture could influence your heart, but if you are pulling your whole body down most of the day, so you are slumped, with rounded, narrowed shoulders and depressed chest, you make pressure inside your chest cavity. Nothing likes being squashed – including your heart. Your ribcage protects this delicate organ – but if your ribcage itself is stiff and immobile because of poor posture, you make things harder work for all your internal organs.

# Further refinement

People who have practiced directed thinking for a period of time become skilled at it, just as you become more accomplished when repeating any skill. My experience of my own process of learning, practicing and refining directed thinking over an extended period of time – in my case three decades, and teaching it to others and training other people to teach it to others – has given me an overview of this skill from many different perspectives. With practice the body itself is thinking. When this happens your brain drives your body from A to B, and your muscle, bone and sinews become more alive. You might call this being in touch with your body, but once again it's a two-way process and your body is in touch with you. This is so different from using your body unconsciously – often just to carry your head around! This state is familiar to experienced musicians, singers, actors and performers who need and work for an interconnectedness of body and mind in order to practice their craft.

# Chapter 3
# Keys to better posture

**This chapter covers:**
- core muscles
- postural unity
- posture informs movement
- How movement starts with our reactions
- How reactions require thought

## Working with new ideas to improve posture

How do you work with new ideas to improve your posture? In this chapter we look at where and how you start exploring your awareness and the unique considerations for postural unity, and why it is relevant to all activities. Of course, it's not as simple as following a series of instructions; your thinking and awareness skills need some attention too. Exploring mental aspects of preventing bad postural habits and encouraging positive ones improves awareness, and helps you challenge your preconceptions about movement and how it starts.

Posture is the precursor to movement, and all movement, whether large or small, starts as a body reaction we make to a stimulus we receive. Our reaction, the things we do, is largely the same, whatever the stimulus. This is good news because it tells us our reaction pattern is something we can

understand and work with. This reaction pattern gets fixed in our bodies and becomes our posture. Before going more deeply into this reaction, find out what you think posture is with this quiz.

## Quiz: test your postural knowledge and beliefs

We all have ideas about what posture is and how to improve it. Test yours by answering these questions – prizes include better knowledge and understanding. This is a simple quiz consisting of a statement and your choice of true or false in reply. Get a piece of paper and jot down your answers – or carry them in your head and then add up your score. You get one point for every correct answer.

### Questions
1. I need core strength to support my posture. True or false?
2. A lumbar support cushion will help my back. True or false?
3. Standing up straight is a sign of good posture. True or false?
4. I need to work on different muscle groups to improve my posture. True or false?
5. If I feel comfortable when driving or sitting then everything is okay. True or false?

6. Exercise will improve my posture. True or false?
7. You can change your posture just by thinking. True or false?
8. Some people naturally have better posture than others. True or false?
9. I inherited my bad back so I have to live with it. True or false?
10. Active rest practice is the single most useful thing I can do for my posture. True or false?

## Answers

1. I need core strength to support my posture. This is FALSE. It is a persistent belief that core strength will give you better posture. Usually people exercise what they think are core muscles, abdominals mostly, in the hope of a better posture. If you do abdominal crunches the most likely thing you'll end up with is a crunched abdomen, and probably a sore neck in the process. Lengthening does more for your posture.
2. A lumbar support cushion will help my back. Sorry – it won't. You will end up compressing your back into it or compressing your back to get away from it. Lumbar cushions attempt to do the work your own back should be doing. So this is FALSE.
3. Standing up straight is a sign of good posture. Not really. Although it's true that slouching and round shoulders are a sign of poor posture, you don't want to be ramrod straight either. People who impose straightness on themselves do so with tension. So again this statement is FALSE.
4. I need to work on different muscle groups to improve my posture. FALSE. Your body is more intelligently organized than that. Think of all your muscles being like a suit, rather than different groups, and you are already thinking more accurately.
5. If I feel comfortable when driving or sitting then everything is okay. Comfort is not always a sign that all is well – our senses can deceive us. We can feel superficially comfortable when driving, but by squashing our inter-vertebral discs and digestive organs. So the statement is FALSE.
6. Exercise will improve my posture. Sadly this is FALSE. If you continue to use your body badly, no amount of exercise will improve your posture – you'll just exercise your bad habits – and get better at them.
7. You can change your posture just by thinking. TRUE. Learning to direct, which is a thought initiated skill, can improve your posture, awareness and body use.
8. Some people naturally have better posture than others. TRUE. Some people do naturally have better posture and body use than others, but everyone can learn to make the best of what they are.
9. I inherited my bad back so I have to live with it. FALSE. You may indeed have an inherited problem to cope with; scoliosis often runs in families. But you can learn to use yourself well and don't have to end up with a bad back simply because a parent has one.
10. Active rest practice is the single most useful thing I can do for my posture. TRUE. Practice regularly to gain enormous benefits. For a full description of active rest and variations, see Section 2.

## How did you do?

- 10 out of 10. You are a postural genius and don't need to read any more. Please give this book to a more posturally challenged friend.
- 7–9 out of 10. Not bad, perhaps you have some ideas you could re-examine.
- 4–6 out of 10. What can I say? Read on and discover lots of interesting ideas to help you.
- 0–3 out of 10. No comment.

# Your core muscles

What makes your muscles strong – and do you need strong muscles to support your posture? Obviously if you are relatively fit, your muscles might be considered strong – or at least strong enough to hold you up as you walk around. But what muscles are needed or used to hold you up? Not necessarily those you think, or even a specific set of muscles. Many unhelpful assumptions have been made about core stability, particularly in relation to helping low back pain and musculoskeletal problems. These assumptions have become beliefs and readily accepted without question. However, it is helpful to look at what you believe and ask yourself if this belief is helpful – let alone accurate. Common assumptions include the idea that certain muscles are more important than others for stabilization of your spine, and weak abdominal muscles lead to back pain. This leads on to the assumption that strengthening abdominal or trunk muscles can reduce back pain.

Another idea about core stability is that there is a unique group of core muscles working independently of other trunk muscles, and having a strong core will prevent injury, because there is a relationship between stability and back pain. Actually, your muscles are more intelligently designed than that, and don't have a 'core' that does all your stabilization. It's more of a synergy of all your muscles, rather than just one set that gives you the ability to remain upright and move around. Some individuals are born without some core muscles, or the deep muscles are fused to other muscles. This is considered a normal variation – just like having an extra lumbar vertebra, and certainly doesn't stop people walking and moving.

During pregnancy abdominal muscles undergo dramatic elongation, and most pregnant women can't do sit-ups (even if they want to), whereas non-pregnant women generally can perform sit-ups – but there is no correlation between whether you can do sit-ups or not and possible backache.

Pregnancy can be a time when women suffer back pain, but this commonly resolves very soon after delivery, well before those stretched abdominal – or core – muscles have returned to their pre-pregnant state. And all post-delivery women have slack abdominal muscles, so why don't they all have a collapsed spine too? Perhaps the role of core abdominals to prevent or cure back pain needs a bit more thinking about. This calls into question the whole concept of abdominal exercises specifically for back pain, or even for good posture.

One other point is the whole idea of tightening certain groups of muscles in order to support yourself. This is almost impossible to maintain for any length of time. One example is being asked to tighten the buttocks of your supporting leg as you walk. This means doing a continuous buttock dance, one buttock after the other, while you walk. Try it – see how far you get. There is a better way.

This is not to suggest that you allow everything in you to be floppy and give up any form of exercise. Exercise has many benefits, but you can increase both the benefits and your enjoyment of movement if you get your posture sorted out as a priority. Read on!

# Postural unity – your primary control of movement and body use

To change your posture you need to think about yourself globally, rather than in bits. It always helps to have a broad brushstroke outline to return to over and over again. Then you can explore all the details, and see how they fit into the bigger picture. In this way, you can set up simple thinking and body use patterns for yourself. When it comes to our posture we have the challenge of organizing our balance over our two feet,

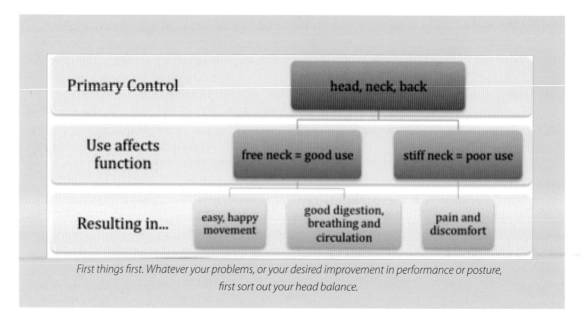

*First things first. Whatever your problems, or your desired improvement in performance or posture, first sort out your head balance.*

usually in motion. This is a complex task, with many factors to take on board; it is so complex that many scientists devote their entire lives to the study of human locomotion and attempt to recreate it in robots, not terribly successfully, but it is a subject of intense scrutiny simply because of its complexity – how do we do it? Fortunately for us most humans find walking easy once learned, and some people can manage excellent posture without thinking about it at all.

If you have an easy structure, no injuries and an undemanding life then you are indeed lucky. Most of us are not so fortunate, and need to address our posture if we want to improve. The problem is – how? What do we do? What should we consider and what should we avoid doing? One of the keys to good posture is to encourage a springy length throughout your whole body, and the most important aspect of length is having a well-organized relationship between your head, neck and back. This should be one of smooth harmony. This harmony (or lack of) will influence the use of the whole of your body and all its functions, such as breathing, digesting and circulation. If this relationship is in disharmony, it will influence all these things for the worse and not the better.

This unique relationship can be considered the primary control of your movement and body use, and it's about how your head balances on your spine. It's primary because it is the broad brushstroke that needs your consideration as a priority; it's the most important thing. If you really want to improve your posture, for whatever reason, you have to consider this vital relationship sooner or later. If you make it sooner, you will get your benefits much more quickly. If you dive straight into trying to sort your posture out, perhaps with exercise programs, you will run into trouble if you haven't sorted out what's going on in your neck and how it's affecting your head and the rest of your torso. On the other hand, getting this relationship smooth and harmonious then makes any exercise you wish to undertake not only easier to perform, but more effective too. It comes back again to thought–posture–movement. Learn the skills of directed thinking so as to influence your posture and movement will follow naturally.

# The listening posts of posture

As upright creatures our head has a great deal of freedom and range of movements that allow us to look around with ease, see where we are going and change direction whenever we wish. Our heavy head balances on a slender neck column quite nicely, or at least, it is designed to do so. Our head sits on the first neck bone, which is called the atlas. This wonderful balancing bone is named after the mythological Greek god Atlas, whose punishment for a misdemeanor was to hold the weight of the heavens on his shoulders, so as to hold apart heaven and earth. Obviously he made a fairly good job of it as they are still keeping their places! We often think Atlas's task was to hold the weight of the world, rather than the sky. As the world is a globe, and our head is a globe supported by a ring shaped bone underneath it, that bone inherited a god's name.

Your atlas bone serves to balance the weight of your head and keep it apart from the rest of your neck and spine. It forms one half of a vital joint, which allows you to nod your head. The other half of the joint is above the atlas bone; it is the base of your skull, the occiput. So this joint is termed the atlanto-occipital joint – but it's easier to think of it as the nodding joint. This joint is like a pivot, but there is more boney weight in front of the joint than behind it. This means something has to be done to stop your head falling forwards all the time – as it does when you 'nod off' when falling asleep in an upright position.

There are layers of muscles and ligaments that join the head to the top neck bones and these all help to keep your head upright so you can see where you are going. The deepest of these muscles lie right next to the bones and are called the sub-occipital muscles. These muscles are tiny, but powerful in their influence on your posture and movement. To some extent they are part of the body's 'listening' muscles, sensitive to nuances of movement that stretch or compress them, helping to tell your head where it is in space – so you don't fall over. They 'listen' to what you do with your head, including what you do with your eyes, and then tell your brain what's going on.

The rest of your back muscles, which chain their way down your spine and legs, 'listen' to the sub-occipitals and respond to what they 'hear', usually by contracting in order to balance things out in your body and keep you upright and walking. If your habit of life and movement is to hold your neck in a virtual clamp, you affect these tiny muscles in a way that makes them a bit deaf – to carry on the analogy of 'listening' muscles. And, their response is to tense up more just in case they have missed anything important – such as the vital need to duck your head. So, tension breeds tension and affects these listening posts of our posture.

If you want to demonstrate this to yourself try this experiment.

## Find those tiny 'listening' muscles, your sub-occipitals

Sit comfortably in an upright chair and put your hands up on either side of your head with your thumbs just under the back of your skull. Start with your thumbs on the boney bump just behind your ears; this is part of the base of your skull. Now slide your thumbs towards each other about an inch inwards, and slightly upwards. This brings them snuggly under the ridge of your skull. Gently press your thumbs in just a little so you can feel the ridge of the back of your skull. Let your fingers come to rest around your temples and face. Read the rest of the instructions before you continue! Close your eyes.

Now, turn your eyes to the right and left, while your other fingers keep your head from moving. You will feel those little muscles changing shape and tone under your thumbs, as if they swell when you turn your eyes one way or the other. Even when your head is not moving, these muscles are responding to your eye movements. You will find that it is impossible to move your eyes without these muscles moving. They are so fundamentally connected that any eye movement is registered by the sub-occipitals. If you are a tense person you might find your whole jaw moving from side to side as you move your closed eyes. Although you can't (and don't need to) prevent your sub-occipital muscles moving in response to your eye movements, you don't need to move your jaw too.

## Case Study
### Adrian: seeing straight

Adrian suffered from low back and knee pain. When he was 10 an accident almost blinded his right eye. He recovered and adapted well; he can drive, and makes his living with a computer. Posturally he is very twisted; his pelvis swivels one way and his knees swivel the other. Walking through a narrow doorway he often bumps his shoulders or hip on the doorframe. Adrian's posture has adapted badly to the new messages that his brain received from his eyes and consequently he developed muscle twists that caused problems.

Eyesight can affect your balance and posture. We can picture the stooped scholar with thick glasses, but eye problems can have a greater impact when unrecognized. Our eyes are organs of balance; without realizing it we are constantly taking measurements of horizontals and verticals to tell our brains where up and down are. We laugh at a distorting mirror in a fun fair making us lose balance, but don't realize our own eyes might have the same effect!

Through his lessons Adrian learnt to monitor his sense of where 'up' is. For most of us, this is obvious, but if your vision is distorted so is your perception of space. Adrian had attributed his clumsiness to being a clumsy person, but it is a result of imperfect postural coordination. Now that

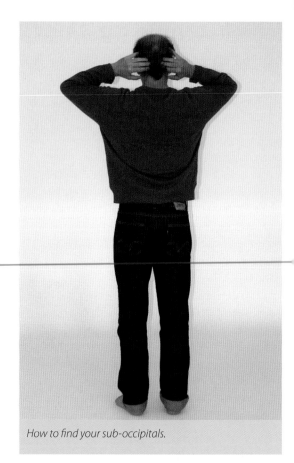

*How to find your sub-occipitals.*

he has a better sense of his body he is much less clumsy – which was an unexpected bonus.

Poor sight can have a profound effect on neck muscles, resulting in a fixing of the neck and head, which has a chain reaction on the muscles of the back and legs. During his lessons Adrian experienced confusion. He felt I had twisted him so he was leaning over, but when I got him to check my full-length teaching mirror he could see this was not the case. His senses were misleading him and he realized he had to stop relying on feelings and work with thinking instead.

Our muscles respond to us giving what Alexander used to call inhibitive and directive orders. Learning to be aware of excessive tension, to cease to engage with it, and to project directive orders to our muscles, is all part of the Alexander Technique.

Adrian's back and knee pain have gone. He can manage his posture and use very well now, catching himself when excessive tension creeps in and taking steps to release it before it builds up.

Here are some tips for eyesight and posture:

- Have your sight checked regularly; your optician will pick up problems.
- Squinting will make you tense your neck. Wear sunglasses in strong light.
- A stiff neck means a stiff ribcage – don't forget to breathe!

## Your head leads, your body follows

When you walk about, you usually navigate with your eyes first. You look to where you want to go, and the action of looking turns your head, which sets off a rotation in your trunk, and takes you round the corner or wherever you want to go. As humans, if we want to we can use even this function in a sophisticated way – looking over our shoulder while we walk in the opposite direction for example, but generally, where your head goes, your body will follow. It's certainly true of a cat that finds itself in the air, after falling the wrong way up so its feet are uppermost. The cat's eyes and inner ear mechanisms will orient its head horizontally. This alerts the sub-occipital muscles, which tone up. The cat's brain 'reads' this piece of information and encourages the spinal muscles to unwind and organize the cat's spine from the neck down, so its feet are under it, ready to land on, before it gets to the carpet. Anyone who has seen a sleeping cat fall off the back of a sofa has seen this little miracle played out – usually ending with the cat walking away nonchalantly, tail waving, pretending nothing happened and it didn't fall at all.

Our head–neck–back relationship functions in much the same way as it does in a cat: the way you use your neck and your head, particularly your eyes, affects the tone pattern for the rest of your back musculature. If you habitually walk with your

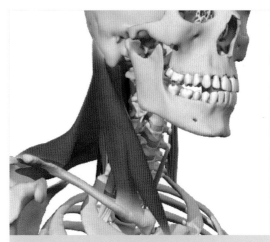

*Neck muscles need tone to support your head, but too much tone turns into tension and effectively deadens the messages that muscles give your brain about movement. So you become stiff and tension builds up.*

head carried on one side, even slightly, it will send a 'twist' message down your back and interfere with your posture and your balance. It may also interfere with your breathing and with free blood flow to your head. So these apparently innocuous habits can have considerable consequences.

## Holding on to your head: the body cringe!

We don't want to lose our heads. Our language reflects the vital role of our head. We admire someone with a cool head, and sympathize with someone who has lost their head in a difficult situation. It usually implies they made a rash decision or an inappropriate action they later regret. When we over-tighten the neck muscles we retract our heads. It's a kind of cringe that starts in your neck and spreads down your back. This response is not only physical but also contains emotional elements. Most animals respond to fear with a retraction of the head, indeed excessive head retraction that exposes the throat is a fear submission gesture from a weaker animal to a stronger animal. I have seen my own dog (which

39

**Do you really retract your head?**
**Try this game with a friend**
This is such a simple demonstration it makes people laugh. All you need is a friend to try it out on, and a pin and a balloon. Look into your friend's eyes and stand quite close, in front of them. Hold up the balloon in one hand, and the pin in the other, in front of their face, at head height. Threaten to bring the pin to the balloon. Your friend will try and get away from the anticipated bang of the imaginary pop! Their neck will stiffen up and they will pull their head back away from the anticipated noise. If you want to, you can do it with an imaginary pin and balloon. It's a powerful little game to try. You may find even reading the description makes you cringe. The physical nature of that cringe is what we are interested in – because that's what you do with your whole body!

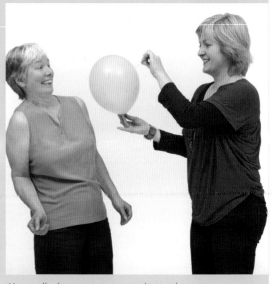

*You really do contract your neck muscles.*

is small) do this in the presence of a larger, more menacing dog. The larger dog usually loses interest at this point, having seen the submission, and my dog can carry on with her business.

Humans also respond to fear – such as loud noises or emotional conflict – by retracting their head on their neck. This retraction then becomes a habit that kicks in before we begin a movement, or builds into a permanent postural state. It becomes part of our movement, an unobserved, but ever-so-damaging habit of being. It is not easy to challenge, being long-standing, but getting to understand your primary control is worth it for the psychological and physical feeling of freedom it brings. A stiff neck makes all kinds of movements difficult, from turning to look over your shoulder to looking up at the ceiling. To find ways of improving your head–neck balance, see the exercises in Section 2.

# Your reactions and why they interfere with posture

Posture comes down to what's happening inside you, your reactions to stimuli. We need stimuli to live. Every living thing needs stimuli. Plants need light, warmth and water and respond to good conditions by growing well. Anyone who has forgotten to water their pot plants can see the consequences of the withdrawal of that particular stimulus. If you have a fast growing plant such as an amaryllis, you know you have to turn it regularly so the light falls evenly on it, otherwise it grows faster on one side than the other and ends up so distorted it is likely to snap under its own weight when the heavy flowers emerge.

What about us? How do we respond to stimuli and why does a poor response interfere with our posture? It comes back to what is going on in your primary control. If you consistently respond to life's big and little challenges by tensing excessively, you will, as Alexander so eloquently described, stiffen your neck, pull your head back and shorten and narrow your back. You might describe this as cringing, exactly what you might do in response to a loud bang. This in turn will deprive you of free flowing circulation to vital organs and make you stressed, grumpy and stiff. You react like this because you have a heavy head on top of a long thin spine; the reaction comes out of your structure and is a common reaction to all mammals with a head and a spine.

Just because it's common doesn't mean it's natural or helpful, and most other mammals let go of the tension pattern once the stimulus has passed, but humans tend to hold on to it. The fact that most people have appalling posture doesn't make it natural or a good idea. It would be easy to blame our over-crowded living for our inner tensions and for squashing ourselves into as small a space as possible, but it isn't really true. You often can't change a stimulus, but you can and should change your response, or at the very least teach yourself to have the choice.

## Posture and stress

There is a direct link between your levels of stress and your posture. A person who is generally relaxed looks easy in their own skin; they also look as if their body is in harmony with itself. Postural stress in this context isn't caused by a specific position but is rather the result of a continuous build up of the poor reactions of your body to the minor and major stresses of your life.

When we think of stress we usually think of something unpleasant that is imposed on us from the outside – perhaps an unexpected bill or a demand made on us by another person. It is easy to believe you might react to that kind of stress badly, but there is a fine line between a stimulus and a stress. In fact, it's so fine a line you can consider any stimulus in the form of stress simply because a stimulus usually leads to a response. And that is where what we commonly consider to

be stress comes in.

Let's say that you walk upstairs badly; you let your body cringe as you ascend the stairs, so your neck is just a bit tight and your head a bit retracted. You probably don't notice it at all or consider it important. But let's say you hold that cringe while you sit at your computer, either working or socializing. And then when you walk out to meet friends, you still carry that cringe in your body. You have hard wired it into yourself and over time it becomes postural stress. It can be subtle so you feel vaguely uncomfortable a lot of the time, or it can be serious enough to suppress your natural breathing pattern and cause you to start hyperventilating because your breathing has become shallow and irregular.

## Case Study
### Martin, 33, stressed and on the edge

Martin has a high stress graphic design job with tight deadlines, which led to him having a tight neck and shoulders. He was constantly on edge and unable to relax. Although only in his early 30s, he was already feeling burned out and bad tempered. He used to work off his stress by thrashing around the squash court, but recently he had suffered a series of minor injuries while playing and finally had to admit this remedy wasn't working – he couldn't drop the stress and couldn't work it off: 'I feel as if it's with me all the time. Why can't I just relax?' he asked me.

So much is said about stress these days, people get confused. Stress makes people perform better according to some researchers; too much stress is bad for you according to others. So what is stress and do we need it? It might be easier to think of stress as a stimulus. We need stimuli of all kinds to react to, in order to function, but if the stimulus is unrelieved and constant, we stop functioning and start to break down. Each of us has a stress level

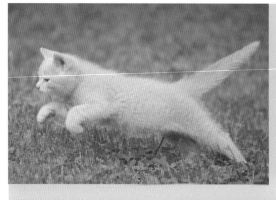
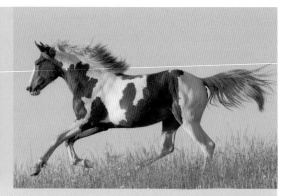
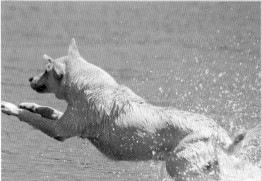
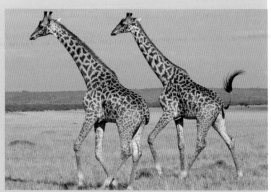

*Whatever the size of mammal, the efficient organization of their heads, necks and backs is vital to their ability to move freely. From kittens to giraffes, the challenge is the same, and so is the response. You can see all these creatures have a forward moving flow of muscular energy throughout their bodies. Even though their spines* *are in the horizontal plane, and yours is vertical, and they have four legs compared with your two, you still want in your body what they have in theirs: a well coordinated flow of muscular support throughout your structure, a freely poised but well-supported head on your neck and a back that offers support for your limbs.*

at which we really work well – we are happy and stimulated – but just a little extra pressure can turn us into harassed, overworked, miserable people who never catch up with themselves.

When Martin started having a glass or two of wine to aid his relaxation he realized he had to change something, but didn't know what or how. He came for Alexander lessons following friends' advice, although he wasn't sure what the Alexander Technique could do for him. He knew it helped with posture, but had not made the link between posture and stress.

During his lessons Martin realized he responded to almost everything in his work and life by

creating a wave of compressed tension through his whole body. This revealed itself in his poor posture; it wasn't just his neck and shoulders but his lower back, legs, even his feet and toes, all held in a deadly grip. He became aware of how much he held his breath, too, and what problems that caused him. He learnt to maintain a sense of lengthening through his back and he practiced lying down with his knees bent and his head supported by books. This helped rebalance the tension in his back and he began to feel more comfortable. He told me that the most useful thing he learnt was how to say 'no' to the excessive work load that had previously been piled on him, because he was now more in touch with his own body and knew when enough was enough.

Here are some comments on and tips for dealing with stress:

- Everyone is different; one person's challenge is another person's overload.
- Tell tale signs of having too much stress include poor sleep, inability to 'switch off', forgetting details and irritability.
- Allow yourself to take time just for you.
- If your shoulders live permanently round your ears and feel tight, chances are you are overstressed!

# Rewire your thinking and posture with inhibition and direction, twin tools for change

You don't want to spend your life in a postural cringe – even a subtle one. Understanding your head, neck and back and how they influence your movement is a good starting point to getting out of the cringe habit, but the next step is discovering some tools that let you use this knowledge (and yourself) in a freer and lighter way. Because we are such strongly driven creatures of habit, it is at habit level we must work.

The most helpful tools we can develop are what Alexander termed inhibition and direction. These are tools that stop our unhelpful reactions to stimuli – the postural cringe that expresses itself in that awful neck stiffening and head retraction, which are our constant companions if we let them – and instead enable us to lengthen ourselves and lighten our muscle loading. These two skills go hand in hand. You can't lengthen if you carry on shortening and there is no point in stopping shortening if you are simply going to collapse in a heap instead. The things we want to stop often start happening well before we realize it; they are so ingrained and automatic that we need to give ourselves time and a quiet situation to observe them. Inhibition and direction make a balancing act in our thinking, one we should pay attention to. It's the best tool for change.

## Take time to stop

For many people the idea of 'stopping' seems very puzzling and irrelevant to their problem. If you have back pain or poor posture — you want to stop the pain or improve your posture, but you have no idea how. What is meant by 'stopping' in this context?

It comes down to unpicking the tangle of our reactions to our situation. If you have poor posture, you will hold your body in a habitual way. If you also have pain of any kind, but particularly back pain, you will hold yourself in a way that minimizes the problem. This 'holding' is your current postural norm, which you do most of the time. You won't be aware of doing it, but you will be stiffening muscles around your back and neck. You will do other things too, such as holding your shoulders rigid, restricting your ribs as you breathe and locking your jaw. All these tensions over stimulate your nervous system, which will make you feel on edge or anxious and jumpy. Even if you move slowly or carefully to avoid pain, your whole system is on the body equivalent of 'red alert' and ready to jump in with even more tension at the slightest movement. This is what you want to stop. The tension quickly becomes a habit and part of your reaction to almost anything, from answering your phone to the act of walking; everything is attempted with excessive and unfelt effort.

Learning to stop this involves learning to take time. For many of us this is an enormous challenge. We live in a 'fix-it' world that leads us to believe that solutions should be quick, if not instant. Our bodies are simply not like that. Whatever caused your postural problems, whether it was a recognized injury, something that came on gradually, or something that happened quickly, your response will have included a clenching right through the core of your being. Learning to 'undo'

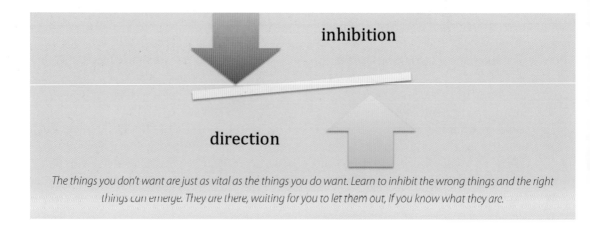

*The things you don't want are just as vital as the things you do want. Learn to inhibit the wrong things and the right things can emerge. They are there, waiting for you to let them out, if you know what they are.*

this takes time. The best place to explore what 'stopping' might mean to you in the active rest foundation position is described in Section 2.

You could easily think this is just relaxation but it's more than that. It isn't about lowering levels of tension, but about finding the appropriate level of tone required for your activity. If you are walking around, you need a lot less effort than you think. If you are engaged in a tug of war then you need a great deal of effort. Our problem is that we unthinkingly bring the same effort to things like cleaning our teeth as we do to a tug of war.

So give yourself time to stop and think about what you are doing and how you move. Do you really need to lock your jaw muscles when you walk up the stairs? Have your shoulders migrated up round your ears as you sit at your desk? What would life be like without those tensions? You'd be calmer, a little taller because tension makes you shrink, and most important you would have learned the value of taking your time.

## Think spiral, not straight lines

If you still think you should be standing up straight, ask yourself what you mean by 'straight'. It's more helpful to consider what you don't want, such as tight muscles and a distorted musculature, than to impose straightness on yourself. There is nothing straight in our bodies. The ends on our bones are rounded; even the long bones of our arms and legs are not straight, they are curved. Our muscles don't go up and down in stripes, they wrap around us in spiral directions. This implies there is a body wisdom we can get in touch with if we know how. When we direct ourselves to lengthen rather than straighten, we could be sitting, standing, curled up in a ball, running for a bus, or practicing active rest. The directed thought lets us undo those things we don't necessarily feel. It offers our whole system a gentle unraveling stimulus that will do the right thing for us if we let it. Like all good things, this is a matter of practice. The more you get familiar with directing in active rest, where there are no demands on you, the easier it is to direct when you are doing something more challenging.

# Chapter 4
# Standing and sitting

**This chapter covers:**

- how to balance on your feet
- how we shorten ourselves
- ways of sitting
- how to sit well

## Balancing on your two feet

When you see people standing still, at bus stops or in shops, their posture reveals how they hold themselves up. If they are springy and light in their body – which is not necessarily related to physical weight – there is little pressure or compression in their spine and joints. This shows in their stance and faces.

Unfortunately a stroll around any park will show you most people have less than optimum posture. A common misuse pattern is a collapsed chest with a rounded upper back and drooping shoulders. The neck is jutting forward and the head retracted on the neck. This puts an unnecessary strain on the neck muscles, which is never relieved because this pattern of head carriage is habitual – it's always there. In order to balance out the jutting head, the knees are often slightly bent and extra weight is thrust into the pelvis and hips. Because the drooping shoulders make the arms uncomfortable, people often either clasp their hands in front of them or put them in their pockets. In this way their chosen posture is balanced out – but at what cost? The distortion of the scaffolding of the body – bones and muscles – is obvious once pointed out, but less obvious is the internal pressure on joints and internal organs.

F. M. Alexander, founder of the Alexander Technique, sometimes called these 'harmful and perverse pressures', and he numbered among his clientele people who suffered as a result, perhaps because of digestive or respiratory problems or constant fatigue. Alexander discovered the use of the body affects its functioning – in other words if you persist in squashing your digestive and respiratory organs because of your poor posture, you can expect those organs to complain and give you trouble.

Our bodies – and minds – work much better when there is internal space. Without it, tension and pressure builds up. We see this clearly in the outside world; a narrow pavement or road often causes a block in the flow of either human or car traffic. If you squeeze a tube of toothpaste, but leave the top on, you can be sure the paste will eventually force its way out – either in a big squirt the moment you take the top off, or finding an escape route through a crack in the tube. Your organs can't do that – they just suffer. Organs are mostly soft tissue and have little resistance to pressure. One of the reasons we have a boney ribcage is to protect vital organs such as heart, lungs and liver. It is literally a cage that saves these

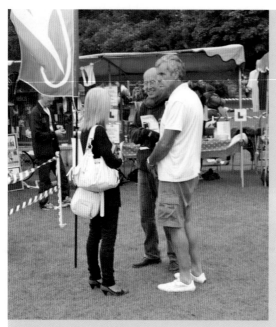 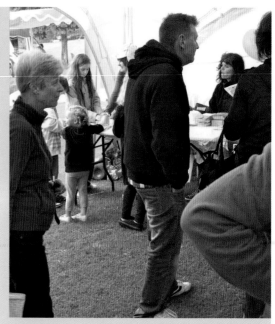

*This is a common misuse pattern. So common we almost think it's natural, but it's not. Collapsed chest, rounded upper back, neck jutting forward and head retracted on the neck. The knees are bent because the pelvis is under pressure from all the misuse in the spine above it and the hands seek to stabilize the posture by*

*being thrust into pockets or clasped in front. This is what is meant by 'shortening in stature.' These people are literally pulling themselves down towards the ground; there is no spring or upright influence in their posture. Their va va has voomed!*

delicate organs from injury and buffeting. But if the cage ceases to be a protector and becomes a jailer, there are problems.

## What goes wrong?

Alexander developed his technique to sort out his own problems. He kept having serious vocal problems, as well as a delicate digestion and constitution. He set out to discover what was wrong with him. His persistence and keen observation skills led him to make his discoveries. He became aware of a shortening that affected his whole stature and was sure this had a bad effect on his voice. He delved further until he discovered exactly what this shortening consisted of, and what he could do about it. What he found not

only solved his voice problems, but improved his digestion and overall wellbeing to a great extent. He also began to realize his discoveries applied to all human creatures and not just himself. The ways we stand, sit and move are all influenced by our basic postural habits. If these habits are unrecognized we are likely to shorten ourselves, and we all do it in much the same way.

## How we shorten ourselves

### We shorten in stature...

Regardless of what activity you are engaged in, your bad postural habits will cause you to shorten in stature. It's easy to interpret this as by shortening neck muscles and pulling our heads back

...and compressing our torso, sometimes distorting our spine...

We shorten in stature...

...and contracting both sets of limbs into our torso...

...so our chest and shoulders are narrowed, and our pelvis and legs tight.

*How we shorten ourselves.*

only applicable to standing up straight, but it's relevant to anything you do. If you are practicing a yoga pose that folds you in half, and your muscle suit is shortened, you won't get the same benefit from your experience that you would get with a lengthened stature. Whether you are riding your bicycle, sitting in the bath, swimming or just eating your lunch, your stature is made up of your coordination of your various body parts. So if you generally shorten, anything and everything you do will require more effort than it needs to.

## ...by shortening neck muscles and pulling our heads back...

Neck muscles are very strong; they need to be because they hold your heavy head in place. They are a bit like guy ropes tethering down a hot air balloon – you need to make sure the tension on all the ropes is balanced if you want to keep the balloon from falling over. If you were to tighten the ropes too much, the balloon would sink into the ground. Your head is not really like a hot air

balloon, but your neck muscles are very much like guy ropes – over tightening them will have an adverse effect on your head and will cause your head to retract, be pulled back and down into your shoulder area. Not what you want.

## ...and compressing our torso, sometimes distorting our spine...

Neck muscles don't stop at your collar area; they go right down your back and blend in with other muscles. Stiffening what you think of as your neck has a compressing effect on your whole spine. This can encourage excessive curvature of the spine. The most obvious symptom of this is an over arched lumbar area where the lower back is pulled inwards towards your front. You might find your front sticks out – no matter how slim you are. Your back also narrows when this happens. Occasionally the compression will be unequal from side to side so your spine gets distorted by the uneven muscle pulls. Many a slight scoliosis is caused by poor postural habits.

## ...and contracting both sets of limbs into our torso...

The muscles of our torso flow out into our arms and legs. When we have compression and shortening in the torso, we also have contraction in our arms and legs. This shows more in the arms, with shortened forearms causing all sorts of problems. Our hip joints, knees and ankles all get fixed by muscles dragging upwards into the torso rather than releasing downwards into their own length. Once more this is true regardless of whether you have your arms and legs straight or bent.

## ...so our chest and shoulders are narrowed, and our pelvis and legs tight

Shoulders are easily disturbed. Their very flexibility means we can distort them without noticing. The most usual distortion pattern is for the shoulders to be over rounded, or permanently raised, often both! Stiff leg muscles cause tense feet. This reduces our connection to the ground and so robs us of useful information about where we are and how our balance is working.

## How we sit

When people come for lessons, they commonly want to be taught how to sit properly. My first response is to say 'sit as little as possible', and my second is to ask 'what kind of sitting?' We do a lot of sitting and it's not a good thing. Often we sit very badly, and for increasing periods of time. Complaints of sore necks, backs and knees from sitting are common. We fail to acknowledge that our general carriage and coordination is important.

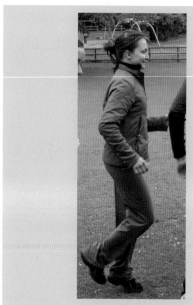

*When we are lengthened, our head is well balanced on the top of our spine and arms and legs are moving freely from a supporting back. With such postural conditions movement is fluid and easy. If you can't stand and walk harmoniously, you won't run harmoniously either. This girl has things working well throughout her structure and is moving easily.*

But we need this for any movement and for the healthy maintenance of our structure, joints, muscles, bones and all our functions. We seem to be far less aware of the effects of our use on our function than previous generations.

I trained in textiles and embroidery many years ago, and my studies included gold work and other church embroidery, and research at the V&A museum. Many old books on embroidery offer considerable advice on sitting to sew, warning that a poor position besides being ungraceful might be injurious to health, and admonishing the would-be embroidery students against the evils of slouching and adopting a cramped attitude or putting their work on their knees. Nevertheless sitting is part of our lives and also a developmental stage in the human child on the journey to independent standing and walking.

A newborn's spine is curved and has no lumbar or neck curve, just one C curve. The first way of exploring its new world is for the baby slowly to gain head control, which starts the development of the neck curve, and this curve increases and assumes its basic shape as the baby practices holding its head up during crawling and sitting. Moving and balancing a relatively heavy head on a slender neck also helps to strengthen muscles of the torso in preparation for future walking, so from an early age sitting is part of what we do, but not for the same reasons that we continue to do it.

# What is good sitting?

If you want to sit well, you have to explore a balancing act. You need to balance your head and your torso, in good harmony with each other, on top of your sitting bones, which are at the base of your pelvis. This kind of balance is not static, but a continuous process, and so good posture and good sitting can't be adequately described in terms of angles or forces – it's more subtle that that.

Balance means movement, and our bodies are designed to move. Even when we think we are completely still, movement is taking place in our bodies. In fact, several things are going on all at once as muscles contract and relax, allowing parts of us to fall and preventing other parts falling. When this works well, we can sit on our sitting bones in easy poise in a springy upright way that is effortless. But if we start to fix ourselves we make this continuous adjustment more difficult; we prevent the ripple of muscle activity that adapts constantly to what we are doing. And instead of being balanced we can start to collapse.

We can collapse much more when sitting than when we are standing and the possibilities of self-inflicted damage to muscles, ligaments and bones is significant – or, as my sewing book said, injurious to health. When we sit well, our muscles are working naturally to support us. Sitting well

is sitting upright with our chest opened out and our balance constantly being made and remade over our sitting bones, so we constantly oscillate in and out of balance from moment to moment. We don't sit bolt upright and still, but move in a way from optimum balance and back into it constantly. These are tiny movements; it doesn't mean you throw yourself around the chair! It always helps to have your feet on the floor as this lets you activate more muscle tone up through your legs, which helps support your trunk and head too, just as it does when you walk. The hallmark of good sitting is that it is easy, and to get it that way requires your attention to the balancing act between your head on top of your spine and your sitting bones at the other end of you. It also requires you to get up, move around and stop sitting as often as you possibly can. If you want to sit well, sit as little as possible.

These are common sitting scenarios:

- sitting at a computer
- sitting to eat
- sitting to drive
- soft sitting, on sofas and soft chairs
- confined sitting, for example on planes or in the cinema

## The harmony of you and the chair

Whatever your sitting situation, you always have to consider the combination of what you're sitting on and how you're sitting. Nearly everyone sits at a computer at some point during the day, and for many people this is a full-time occupation. People put a great deal of thought into the kind of chair they sit in. Should it be an ergonomic chair? Should I have a lumbar support for my lower back? Can I adjust the height? You can spend a great deal of money on the apparently perfect chair and still have problems. These are usually because all the consideration has been given to the chair and none to you as you sit in it. However good your chair, if you want to keep your back healthy you need to get up from it and move regularly and frequently – at least once an hour, preferably more. This means every hour – not just occasionally.

Make a habit of getting up to fetch a glass of water, to talk to a colleague, or simply to stretch your legs and move around a little. As your structure is unique there is no such thing as a good chair; there is only a good chair for you. Be sure that the seat of the chair is parallel to the floor, and has no backward tilt at all. This is to ensure that your hip joints are not under pressure. Be sure that your knees are not higher than your hips when you're sitting. If you have long legs you will have long shins, and when you sit in a standard sized chair it's likely that your hips are lower than your knees. You have to do something about this. You can adjust your position by adding height to your chair seat – a telephone book might do the job. Don't be tempted to use a cushion as you will not get the correct support from it.

When you're sitting at your computer make sure that your feet are flat on the floor. The habit of winding your legs around the legs of the chair or sitting cross-legged creates additional pressure in your lumbar area and abdominal region. If you find that you constantly want to pull your feet under your chair this is likely to be because your legs are habitually tense. This tension then becomes very familiar to you and feels natural, so the desire to tuck your feet back can be very strong. This is one of the most important habits to break. If you get up frequently, you will find it easier to remind yourself that your feet should be flat on the floor when you're at your computer, and particularly when you're typing.

The back of your chair should be either completely upright or slightly angled backwards, but only slightly. Mostly, sit away from the back of the chair so you are not leaning on it. You want your own back to do the work, not the chair back. If you habitually lean on the back of your chair you will do so by pressing into it, creating compression in your back and teaching your muscles that they

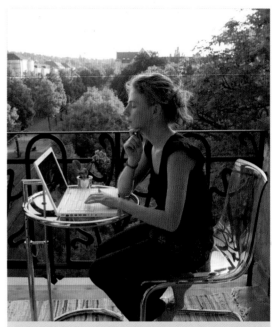

*If you sit like this you have no support in your body, only pressure and compression.*

can't support you. This is a recipe for disaster. If that is the message your chair gives your back, your back will come to rely on the chair to hold it up, and lose useful tone.

There is no harm in leaning back very occasionally. If your back aches without support that is a sure sign you aren't nicely coordinated. If you wish to use the back of the chair, sit well back on the seat so your whole back is in contact with the chair back, not just your upper back.

## The synergy of sitting

Whenever and however you sit, there are three main areas that can come in for a lot of misuse: your sitting bones, hip joints and lower back. These areas affect each other and influence your sitting posture enormously. They also affect your standing and walking posture. Sitting is a good place to consider these areas. If you don't sit on your sitting bones – and the common name of these bones is a big clue to their function – you are likely either to sit heavily on the top of your thighs, causing great compression in your hip joints by doing so, or sit behind your sitting bones, with your lower back curved backwards and intensive pressure in your lumbar spine.

## Find your hip joints and sitting bones

One of the biggest problems people have with sitting is that they don't really know where their hip joints are. The figure below shows how low down the pelvis hip joints are, and their close relationship to the sitting bones at the bottom of the pelvis. These two curved bones are in the middle of your buttocks. Try sitting with your

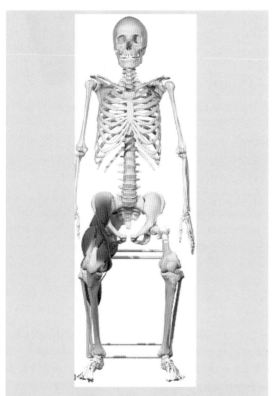

*The skeleton, sitting on his frame box, is well balanced. The sitting bones and feet take the weight and allow the rest of the bones to be in balance. But what happens when you add on all the flesh and the stresses and strains of work?*

fingertips in the middle of one buttock cheek and you will feel them easily. The easiest way to locate your hip joints is to stand up with your legs straight, then pick one leg up with the knee bent. Where did the top of the leg bend? That's your hip joint!

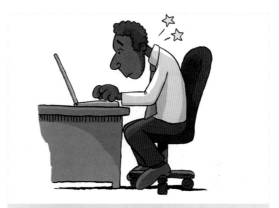

*Ouch! Not the best way to sit.*

## Sitting at a desk

Whether you are sitting at a computer, to read, or in a meeting, your chair needs to have a firm base so your sitting bones have contact with the chair. This in turn allows your hip joints to stay free. If you are not sitting on your sitting bones, you are more likely to create compression in your hip joints as they become part of what has to balance you and hold you reasonably upright. But your sitting bones, with proper contact with a chair, stimulate length through your torso. This, too, is one of the fundamentals of sitting: if you're not sitting on your sitting bones, you are liable to be sitting more towards your sacrum than is desirable. If you sit in this way habitually, the top of your pelvis is liable to tip slightly back. This is why people feel a lumbar cushion or wedge is comfortable, because it pushes the top of the pelvis forward again.

   It would be much healthier if instead of pushing the pelvis back by sitting incorrectly, and then counteracting that with the postural wedge, you located your sitting bones and sat on them. Consider sitting on a large exercise ball, well

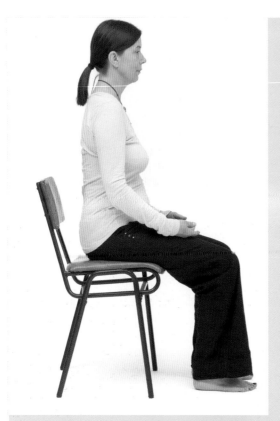 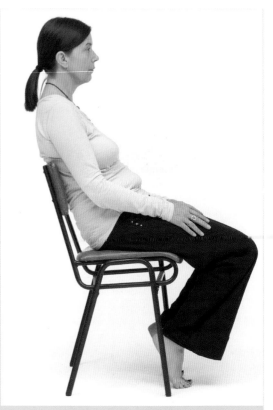

*In the first photo, Jane shows balanced sitting, just like the skeleton in the previous photo. Her feet are flat on the floor; her knees and hips are in a good relationship to each other; her back is upright without effort; and her head is nicely poised on the top of her neck. She is sitting on her sitting bones and so can free her hip joints.*

*In the second photo Jane has allowed her back to collapse against the back of the chair, and tucked her feet back. Without the support from the floor, her body*

*weight is concentrated in her hips and lower back, which come under pressure. Her internal organs will also be under pressure and she will be more inclined to breathe shallowly or to resort to absent-minded mouth breathing to take air in easily. Jane is leaning against the back of the chair, which creates further pressure on her upper back although it will initially seem comfortable to her. If you sit like this habitually, your upper back muscles come to depend on the chair and not on you.*

inflated. This has the advantage of ensuring your keep your feet on the floor – or you'll fall off the ball – and in order to keep your balance you have to micro manage your sitting bone contact with the ball. This often means you move in constant small oscillations around your sitting bones in order to keep your balance. As it has no back, you certainly won't be tempted to lean backwards.

When I have a lot of writing to do – for example when I was writing this book – I switch between

sitting on a ball (making sure I frequently pump it up properly) and sitting in a Victorian dining chair with a wide, flat, firmly padded seat and an almost upright back, which I don't lean on. I always have water close by – in my case in a bottle so I'm less likely to drench my Mac. I drink little and often, which naturally results in visits to the bathroom, and so I move. If I am working to a deadline, I set a timer for every half hour and make myself get up – regardless of how fast I perceive this deadline

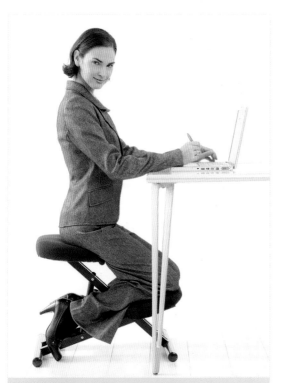

*Do you really want your lower back pulled forward like this? It puts you under constant strain. Notice the tense look about this woman's neck, too. Whatever you do in one part of your back affects the rest of it. The two most vulnerable areas are your neck and lower back, simply because they are not attached to your ribs and so are free to move and therefore be misused.*

to be approaching. I build in mini semi-supine breaks, lying on my back on the floor with my knees bent and my head resting on some books (this will be explained in detail later), and switch my seat from ball to chair every time I take my break. This way I stay fresh, I can concentrate and I end the day feeling supple and relaxed. Without the breaks I stiffen up, my breathing becomes shallow as I concentrate, I become a little oxygen depleted and start to panic, and I get irritable with my nearest and dearest – and myself. It just doesn't work.

## Meet my chair

This is the most comfortable chair I've ever found. A firm, wide, padded seat gives me plenty of space for my long thighs, and the padded back offers just a little support when I lean back for a moment or two of reflection. Another reason this chair is good for me is it is heavy: I can't tilt it onto two legs and disturb my balance, and I can't twist it around, so if I want something I have to stand up and go and get it. The chair stays where it is and I do the moving.

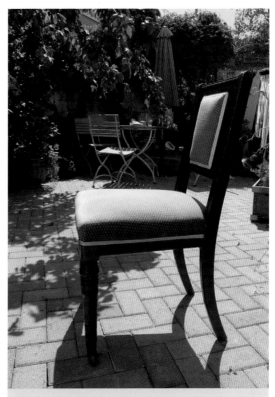

*My chair.*

## Sitting and eating

When you eat at a restaurant, you are at the mercy of the chairs provided and the best you can do is not succumb to the shape the chair wants to make you, and keep a sense of lengthening through your upper back. If there is a choice of chairs, look for one with a level seat as the most important

53

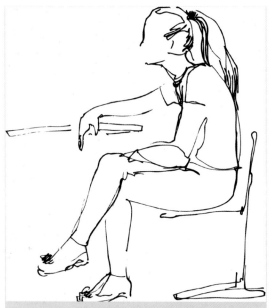

*Bon appétit! How do you think your digestion will cope with this posture?*

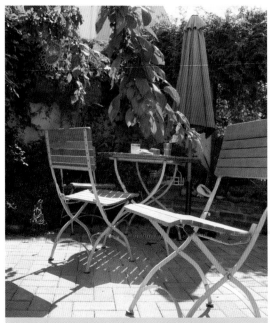

*Comfortable? No, it won't be. The shape forces you to lean back and push your upper back onto the chair back. Your hip joints will be squashed; so will your digestive system. Sitting in this type of chair to eat is stressful.*

thing. Avoid sitting on low sofas and eating off a low table. This seems to be a 'casual' option offered in some pubs. It isn't comfortable and it isn't good for your posture. If you suffer from back pain and eat out regularly it is worth having a firm triangle-shaped wedge cushion that makes whatever seat you are confronted with flat. You can make sure the chairs you eat in at home are suitable. Avoid those with bucket-shaped seats, or dips supposed to fit your bottom – they won't! Look for something simple with a flat seat and a more or less upright back, just as you would for sitting and typing. If you like eating outside and are buying patio furniture, watch out for the tipped back seats, where the front of the seat is higher than the back. They are very common and put a strain on you, as you have to pull yourself forward to the table in order to eat your lunch.

## Driving

If you drive, it is worth giving a lot of thought to your driving position. As always you need to find the right combination of your body and the seat. If you have a long back, you may find the ergonomically designed car seat supports you in all the wrong places. Most seats tilt you too far backwards in order to get your feet on to the pedals. You can end up almost as if you are lying in a hammock. This will have the effect of putting a lot of pressure on your lumbar area as you sink into your pelvis and lower abdomen, and can lead to back pain. Start with adjusting your seat so the back is more upright; if the seat pad is adjustable ensure it is the correct height from the floor for your legs, so you can easily reach the pedals without strain. With the seat back more upright you might find you want to adjust the distance from the steering wheel. Your arms should be close

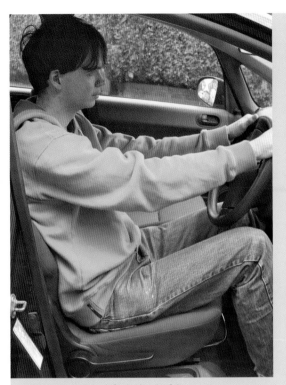 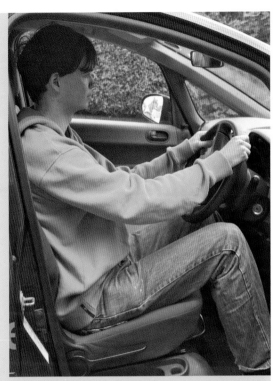

In the photo on the left, the back of the seat is too obtuse, so it is leaning too far back. Being tall, this young driver has adapted by collapsing his chest and upper back so he is pressing into the seat. This encourages his neck to be under pressure and his arms to stiffen. Driving like this for any period of time will be very tiring and stressful. This is a very common situation and will lead to bad postural habits both inside and outside the car. It is more difficult to turn your head when it's held in this way, so over a period of time, neck pain builds up and head rotation become more difficult. Reversing then becomes difficult as you can't turn and look over your shoulder easily. In postural terms, there is no spring in the driver's body, and no useful direction through his back; his head is pulling back on his neck and he is shortening. This is visible in the driver's upper body, if you know what to look for, but the inner tension levels and the stiffness of his legs, which follows on from a shortened posture, are not obvious.

In the photo on the right, a more upright seat back has enabled the driver's back to support him better. There is no pressure on his neck or shoulders, he can breathe easily and concentration will be no problem. The driver's back can lengthen so his shoulder girdle is supported properly by his rib cage. Everything is better balanced in his body. The combination of the correct seat position for him and his own internal direction give him the best driving conditions.

enough so you can have a bend in your elbows with your hands in the correct 'ten to two' position. You shouldn't need to pull your shoulders forward to achieve this.

As well as finding the optimal set-up, consider your personal tension levels, which are largely influenced by your habits. No matter how good your car seat is, if you drive around with excessive tension in your neck, your head will retract and create further pressure through your neck, shoulders and back. It will also affect your breathing, making you breathe in a shallow manner. This in turn will make you more anxious, and affect your concentration, which is affected by anxiety. You may feel you are hyper alert whereas in fact you are over anxious and more likely to make an error of judgment.

## Case Study
### Sara, nervous driver

Sara found driving frustrating. The constant traffic, the road works and the unfair speed cameras all contributed to a stressful experience. She summed it up: 'I find myself gripping the steering wheel so tightly my fingers go white. And since having my lessons I notice that I arch my back away from the seat, I'm so tense.' I asked Sara to mimic holding the steering wheel while she was having her lesson, and she brought her hands up and immediately stiffened her neck so much I was surprised it didn't cause her immediate pain, but she hadn't noticed. Along with the stiff neck, Sally clenched her jaw and held her breath. When I gently pointed these things out to her she was shocked: 'And I'm only pretending; it will be much worse when I'm really driving won't it?' she cried.

Fortunately there are ways you can help yourself when driving. First, acknowledge that you are one of those people who find driving stressful; second, accept that you can't change the traffic, the road

works or the speed cameras, but you can change the tension levels that build up in you. It doesn't matter what has caused you to get tense, it will always affect you in your neck and reveal itself in your breathing. These two elements together will make you stiffen your back as well, which is one reason why some people get back pain from driving.

Releasing tension in your neck muscles is a matter of practice, and you won't be able to do it while driving if you don't practice outside the car! Sara realized that she already had skills she could use. She practiced active rest every day and could encourage her back to lengthen and her neck to release. She then transferred her skill of release to her driving and was very pleased with the result.

She felt much less tense, less anxious and more confident. She told me she had been changing her route home from work to avoid a difficult right turn. She had been nervous and often got beeped by impatient drivers behind her, which made her even tenser. Now she was able to wait patiently until the traffic permitted her to turn right without getting anxious, and when other drivers honked their horn she simply ignored them and didn't let the honking make her rush out into the fast moving traffic.

After each lesson Sara had to adjust her driving mirror because she had lengthened so much, then gradually over the next week she pulled down again. When she realized this, she recognized the amount of tension she brought to driving and was able to deal with it.

## Soft sitting: the dreaded sofa

Ah, the comfy sofa. It grabs you in its squashy arms and holds on to you. Most sofas have a very deep seat – longer than the average thigh – and the seat tips up at the front so you are encouraged to sit back in it, but it's a struggle to get out of it. There is no support for your sitting bones, unless you have a lovely, old-fashioned, very firm leather Chesterfield. Add a TV dinner and you're well on the way to postural hell. If you have sat at a computer all day, driven to and from work, eaten your lunch at your desk or sat in the canteen you are likely to be feeling tired and wanting to flop on the sofa. You are better off enjoying a few minutes of active rest to rebalance your energies. If you can choose your sofa, go for one with a high back and a shorter, flatter seat.

## Confined sitting, planes and cinema seats

If you suffer from back pain, you may be apprehensive about traveling, particularly flying. Most forms of travel involve sitting for extended periods of time and this can give rise to cramp and additional stiffness, and aggravate back pain. There are skills you can use to help in these situations.

First of all you have to be realistic – if you have severe back problems a long haul flight is best avoided unless you have no choice, but preparing physically for a shorter journey can decrease the problems. Make sure you start your journey in a good state. Doing some active rest before you leave the house helps you be more aware of when you are starting to slump and cause compression in your back and joints. Breathing is another consideration. Travel is stressful even if you enjoy it, and when you are stressed, you tend to hold your breath and your breathing becomes very shallow. This will make it more likely that you will compress your ribcage and so put pressure on your digestive organs. Combine this internal pressure with plane food and you can end up with indigestion as well as back pain.

There are simple tools you can use to make your journey more pleasant. If you are flying for any length of time remember that you are likely to swell a little bit because of inactivity, so don't wear tight clothes, particularly not tight jeans as they will feel tighter and tighter as the journey goes on – most uncomfortable. Take advantage of any opportunity to lie down in active rest, so choose a good book you can read on the plane or put under your head when you lie down. People do all sorts of things in airports so no one will notice.

Get up from your seat at any and every opportunity, which will annoy the air stewards, but they don't have your back pain! Give yourself a posture awareness workout for five minutes every hour: attend to your back and ask it to lengthen; ask your neck to release any residual tension; and let your head go up to the roof of the plane. Check your breathing and enjoy moving your ribs. Don't sit still, but wriggle to help protect you from getting cramp. Wriggle your ankles, knees and pelvis. Do a little buttock dance, shifting from one sitting bone to the other and back again. Drink water. Dehydration affects your back as well as making you feel sluggish. Your discs need fluid to maintain their cushioning abilities; if your body lacks water the discs will tend to compress and add to back ache. For the same reason avoid drinks that stress your body, such as coffee or alcohol. Choose fruit juices and dilute them with water instead.

## Sitting to play a keyboard

If your sitting is vital to you to play the piano or organ, you need to be able to move freely about the keyboard and vary the pressure you use to play to get the shades and tones you want. This demands not only musical knowledge and ability, but hours of practice too. If that practice has been carried out with poor posture, you have practiced that too and it will give you problems sooner or later. Posture is of particular interest to pianists because it influences the free movement of the arms and fingers so much. Many pianists have difficulty with their breathing, particularly if they are accompanying a singer and need to listen closely to the performance. While they are listening, they often forget to breathe and so end up stiff and tense.

## Case Study
### Ross's story

Take Ross, who was getting cramp in his forearms and muscle pain in his upper arms after periods of playing. He had always been told that his posture was poor, but had no way to improve it apart from trying to sit up straight. He couldn't maintain himself in this position for very long and inevitably slumped down after a few minutes.

When he was younger he didn't notice any effects of his posture and thought his piano teachers nagged him about his sitting posture just for the sake of appearance. In recent months, the pain started and has got worse. Now he has to consider what to do for the best.

Through working with balanced sitting, Ross began to realize the importance of getting his back muscles to support him while sitting. This meant knowing where his head was aiming, rather than letting it drop towards his music. He soon discovered for himself the Alexander principle that the head leads and the body follows. Most people think this is just to do with movement, but it is also to do with the orientation of the whole body while being relatively still.

This orientation of the body upwards encourages the ribcage to be nicely poised. This in turn provides a proper platform for the shoulder girdle to rest on. This is crucial to any free movement of the arms and fingers because if the ribs do not support the shoulder girdle from below, we hang on to it from above with the neck muscles and give ourselves all sorts of problems.

Ross found he could release excess tension in his upper arms, too, once his sitting was better organized. He is pain free now and delighted to have survived the grueling demand of playing for a summer school, a full eight days of intensive work.

Tense shoulders always lead to a tense neck; get balanced over your sitting bones for ease of movement.

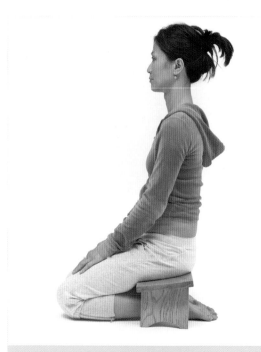

*Your pelvis remains upright on a posture stool, encouraging an upright spine.*

## The posture stool

A simple way to improve your posture when sitting is to spend a little time each day on a posture stool. This is similar to a meditation stool except it is a fraction higher. The stool seat is very slightly angled so your sitting bones are automatically well placed. This makes it almost impossible to collapse your lumbar spine as your pelvis remains upright on your sitting bones. The stool promotes an upright back in a very easy way. You can watch TV, read or simply sit on this stool.

# Chapter 5
# Posture and pain

**This chapter covers:**
- head balance
- neck injuries
- back pain
- self help for your back pain
- posture and breathing

## The crucial relationship

The coordination between your head, neck and back is crucial to understand if you want to improve your posture. The best way to think about it is to consider what you are doing with your torso, and how your head balances on the top of your neck as it emerges from your torso. If you choose open shoulders and a compression free back, your neck and head are well supported and your arms and legs can move freely and easily. How you organize support for your neck and head is the outcome of what you are doing with your torso, and in turn influences how well you coordinate your torso. It's a reciprocal relationship. To put it another way, the carriage of your head is very important. If you wish to improve your posture to help your back or neck pain, work with this relationship.

## The rogues' gallery

The figures on pages 60–61 are from my rogues' gallery of heads that have lost their direction. Every one of them is badly supported. In some cases they are barely supported at all; in others the incredible neck tension has so distorted the delicate neck vertebrae they have either been squashed into curvature or the whole neck column has been dragged forward. Some of the pictures are of people having their posture assessed and others are of the great British public about its daily business. The way you carry your head in daily life is the most significant thing about your posture. It's not what you're doing when you are trying to create a good impression – or to straighten yourself up – it's about what you are doing unthinkingly and habitually. Some people are standing, others walking or sitting. In every case you have to support your head. So the question is, how are you wearing your head? If you recognize yourself in my rogues' gallery, it's time to take action.

## Happy head gallery

The figures on pages 62–63 are from my happy head collection. They are people doing a variety of things, some stressful, some not. They all show poise and balance. It's not so much that these people are aligned properly, but the relationship between their head and their neck is an easy one, not a damaging one. If you carry your head like this, you are well on your way to good posture.

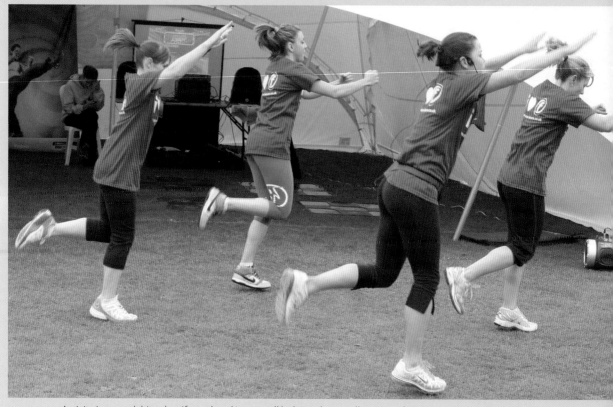

*Activity is a good thing, but if your head is not well balanced, you will move with compression in your body. All movement has to start with consideration of your posture before you start strutting your stuff.*

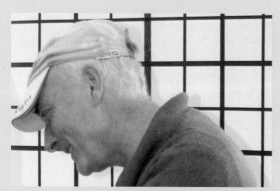

*Years of a dropped neck have increased the rounding in the upper back so it is now a permanent fixture. It's never too late to start undoing it though!*

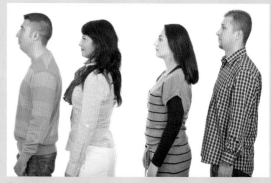

*Each person in this posture line up shows a poor head balance and its effect on their back and posture. All of them are holding their necks stiffly. Even though they are looking forward and trying to stand upright, they wouldn't win any posture prizes.*

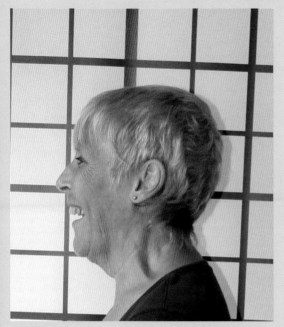

Neck tension has shortened and almost crushed this neck and the sterno-cleido muscles (running from behind the ear to the collar bone) are so tight they stand out.

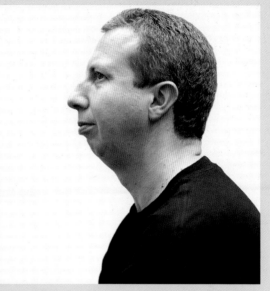

This is a classic 'head forward' posture. The man's neck is dropped forward well in front of his shoulders and he has compensated by pulling his head back, which is why the back of his neck looks so short. Downwards compression in his neck has created jaw tension, too, and his head is locked at the 'nodding' joint.

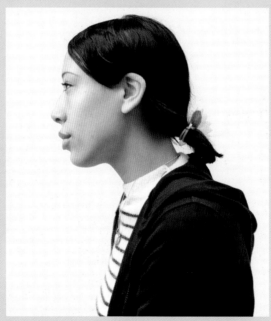

This young woman already demonstrates the same dropped neck pattern of misuse, sometimes called 'text neck'.

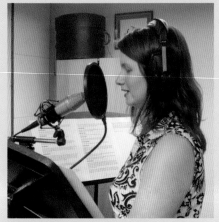

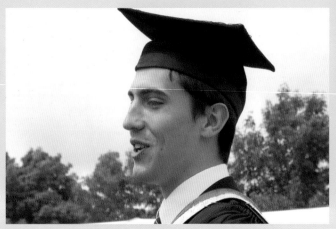

Despite heavy headphones and being in a recording studio reading a script, this is a happy head nicely balanced on the neck without compressing it.

Happiness is having a well-balanced head on your shoulders.

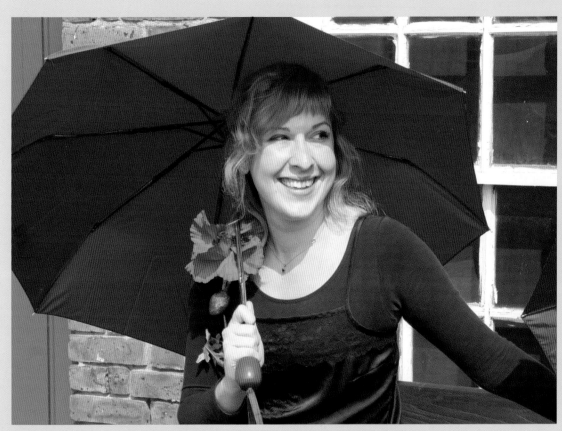

Good head balance isn't about holding yourself artificially straight; it's about having the freedom to move easily, turning your head as you wish. This is a vital skill for actors.

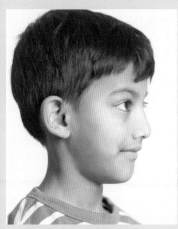 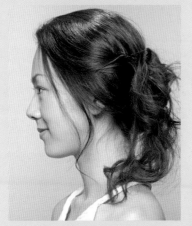 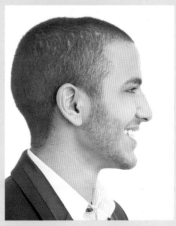

*Happy heads are balanced on well-supported necks, which are long at the back and front. The top joint (nodding joint) is not jammed and everything below the neck, in the torso and legs, will be equally free. This is good postural organization.*

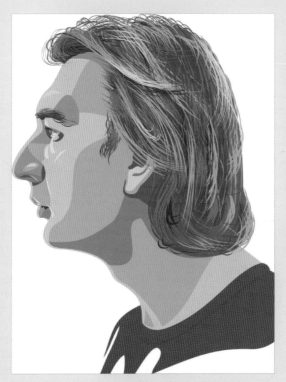

*This misuse pattern is so common it is accepted as normal and even cartoon characters suffer from it. Look how far forward from the man's upper back his neck and head are – too far! This pattern also creates pressure on the vocal apparatus housed inside the throat. Many vocal problems have their roots in postural misuse, as Alexander discovered.*

Notice these people look confident and not tense. They seem relaxed even though they may be engaged in something demanding, like a recording session or acting. It's not about what you do; it's all about how you do it.

# Neck injuries

Sometimes neck problems are a result of an accident rather than postural misuse. In situations like this, the accident can have a profound effect on postural balance and it is the compensation pattern that you make which causes a continuation of pain and problems. This can get into a vicious cycle where pain causes yet more compensation, compensation causes pain, and it all spirals round and round. Whiplash is a common neck injury following a car crash. It can leave residual damage that causes tension that is difficult to resolve. This in turn can lead to stress, which is often accompanied by shallow breathing, which in its turn often makes you mentally foggy. Here is one woman's story of a neck injury that prevented her from practicing her career and caused her much pain and misery.

## Case Study
### Dolores, physiotherapist

I am a physiotherapist and I love my work. I enjoy helping people and believe the best way to do so is to have good conditions in your own body.

Four years ago I had a serious car accident. As a result, I needed orthopaedic surgery and had a metal plate attached to three cervical vertebrae and two intra-vertebral discs replaced in my neck. After a tough year of convalescence, I thought the worst was past, and was very excited gradually to begin to get back to my normal life and activities. Normal life for me was my passion for my

profession and enjoying physical activities in my free time.

But the worst had not passed and I endured one more year of daily suffering, trying to recover neck mobility and relieve the constant pain. It was awful to bear such a level of pain after each day of work or physical activity. I managed to overcome some of the pain thanks to treatments from my colleagues and physiotherapy professionals, and especially with the help from my teacher in myofascial release.

Three years passed since the accident, and I told my myofascial teacher I was a completely different person thanks to his help; I had improved a lot and had enough energy to lead my life. But I still needed his help to stay at that level of wellbeing. I told him how tired and frustrated I was by reading and studying all kinds of disciplines as I looked for a solution to my problems. I wanted to be able to find the precious physical and mental wellbeing for myself; I am the kind of person who believes that the only way to give the best help to others is to have wellbeing characteristics in yourself. Unfortunately I lost all of that after the accident.

My teacher suggested it might be interesting for me professionally and personally to try a different approach – the Alexander Technique – to help with my posture and my pain. I didn't hesitate, and tried a few private lessons. I will never forget the feeling of freedom and wellbeing I experienced in that first session. It seemed more mental than physical.

What happened? I didn't understand the process that brought me that relief, but I clearly felt I was touching a possible solution, so I decided I wanted to explore this experience and I began training at Carolyn's school in Brighton. Each day of training, I reaffirmed that I was developing a more appropriate response to reconnect with my wellbeing, where I could learn skills for myself. I finished my first year of training and resumed my work as a physiotherapist. How wonderful it was to discover myself, finally, helping and caring for others without feeling any pain or emotional fatigue after a busy day.

With the Alexander Technique I have finally learned how to reconnect, experience and develop the maximum wellbeing not only physically, but also emotionally. My neck is pain free and I can move with ease.

# Your back pain

Nearly everyone suffers from some degree of back pain at some point in their life. I've never met anyone who has never had even a twinge, and I've met a lot of people whose back pain has ruled their life. There are so many causes of back pain and so many different ideas on how to cure it that it's easy to get confused and despondent. Don't worry, this book isn't about preaching yet another wonder method, it's about understanding a little of the mechanics of your back and how you might use that understanding to your advantage. If you think of your back as a delicate, finely tuned tool, it will make sense to you that you want to use that tool properly. That is what this book is about.

## What kind of back pain?

Our backs hurt for many different reasons. Everything from a dose of the flu to emotional distress, injuries, overwork, stress and disease registers in our backs. It's always wise to make sure your pain isn't the sign of disease. The kind of back pain sufferer this book is aimed at is someone who lives with it, either intermittently or constantly, and has probably been told at some point that their problems are postural or caused by stress. There are two common categories of pain: acute pain and chronic pain. Most people have experienced both sorts.

## Acute pain

Acute pain usually happens suddenly, when back muscles go into spasm for no obvious reason: 'I just leaned over and something went in my back.' Acute pain can be caused by injury, too, anything from jarring your back by stepping off a step

that wasn't there, or running for longer than your fitness can really cope with, or of course falls, trips and accidents. People can often trace the onset of their years of back trouble to falling down the stairs as a child or falling off a horse or a wall. The acute phase of back pain requires help, and if it is your first such episode you will most likely be in medical care. However, if you are someone who has long-standing chronic pain, which occasionally flares up into acute pain, then your attitude and needs are different.

## Chronic pain

Chronic pain is usually with you most of the time. It may be at a low level or it may be debilitatingly high; sometimes it comes and goes in a seemingly random way. For most people, pain varies from day to day. It's always at the back (or the front) of your mind and you instinctively avoid movements or situations that might set your pain off. This kind of pain is often related to postural habits, or the way your individual body is put together. Investigations often reveal a degree of scoliosis (twisting). The mirror shows you hold one shoulder higher than the other, or a sideways view shows your lower back curving forwards too much.

There are many factors that affect chronic pain, and unraveling the tangle of posture, structure, body use and the influences of your activities, breathing and work is a time-consuming process. Chronic pain is sometimes interspersed with acute episodes. The different elements that operate in back pain reinforce each other. If you have a difficult structure, such as a long back, your posture is poor, you sit all day in your job, and you breathe shallowly you are very likely to suffer from back pain or other problems.

## Your structure

Understanding your structure helps you use it better. Postural improvement starts with awareness of your body. Good use of your body starts with awareness of how you move, sit and are put together. So, let's look at the back, starting

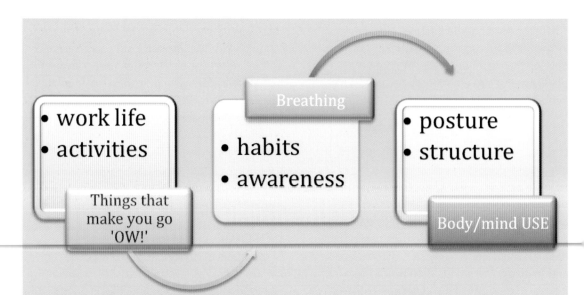

*The relationship between work–life activities and posture*

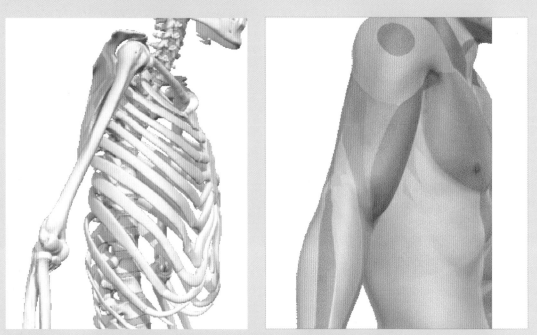

*Notice the curves in the spine; they help absorb shock. If we had a totally straight spine we would be rigid and jar our brains with every step we took, but the curves help us to be more flexible and respond to our body weight hitting the ground as we walk or run. So we don't want a straight, bolt-upright spine – it won't help. On the other hand, if the curves become too exaggerated they don't absorb pressure so well; they become compressed and our spine descends into rigidity, this time in the opposite direction. Actually, it's better to be very upright than collapsed in a heap – but neither is ideal.*

with the inside, your spine.

Think of your spine as a shock-absorbing spring that's deep inside your body. Most of us think of our backs and spines as being near the surface of the skin. We can poke the knobbly bits of our back bone and think, 'Ah, spine!' Actually, it's not easy to decide where your back stops and your front starts, is it? Is there a seam down your side dividing your front from your back? I hope not. Have a look at the picture of a spine opposite and remind yourself that the front of it, the inside if you like, is pretty much in the middle of your torso. The discs are highlighted in green. When you compare it with a fully fleshed torso, it's not so easy to appreciate the depth of the spine, but understanding this one fact about your torso helps you to think about your whole torso lengthening.

## Lengthen your back to improve your posture

One of the most useful things you can do to improve your whole body use is to lengthen your back. This is an easily misunderstood concept. First of all, although I say 'back', a more accurate word might be 'torso', because your back is very much connected to your front. Your ribs, for example, circle their way from your sternum (breast bone) to your spine. Ribs are curvy bones with a great deal of potential spring and flexibility built into their structure, and the fact that they join your back and your front together sheds some light on the idea of lengthening your 'torso' rather than back. But what does this idea of lengthening entail? And how might you set about it?

We have seen how the role of the neck and head play a profound part in posture, and when we consider the 'back' what we are interested in is whether the head, neck and back work as one harmonious whole. This can be misinterpreted as asking, 'Is the head, neck and back in a straight line you could drop a plumb line through?' We tend to make judgments about posture from what it looks like from the outside. When we do

this, we inevitably attempt to sort things out from that perspective. Perhaps we stand in front of a mirror and pull our raised shoulders down, or we attempt to hold our bodies in what we hope is the correct way. This approach takes no account of the internal dynamics of posture, which is the real secret to change. Posture is about relationships of our 'parts' to our 'whole', and lengthening your back is entirely about undoing hidden tensions that shorten it. It is a process of release, not a process of imposing any kind of shape or alignment on yourself. The two photos on page 68 go some way to illustrate this confusion.

## Work life

Posture is a moving, changing balance of your body, and all your activities influence it. If you have a sedentary work life, perhaps sitting at a computer all day, it will have an impact on your posture. If you sit for long periods you put a great deal of strain on your back. The best way you can help yourself is to sit with greater ease and freedom and make sure you get up and move around as much as you can.

## Activities

Just as your work life can cause problems, if you balance it out with an exercise program, but you perform it with poor body use, you will not improve your posture, back pain or whatever else you hope to improve. Instead you are likely to make it worse. This is because you bring to all your activities, whether at work or at leisure, the same pattern of body use. It's your constant personal relationship with gravity. If you respond to gravity in a light, springy way that extends your muscles and lets your spine work like the spring it is designed to be, it doesn't matter what you do. You are less likely to run into trouble with your posture and any injuries. If on the other hand your whole body use is poor and uncoordinated you are more likely to injure yourself, particularly doing something new. If you decide you are unfit and take up running in your effort to get fitter, you are

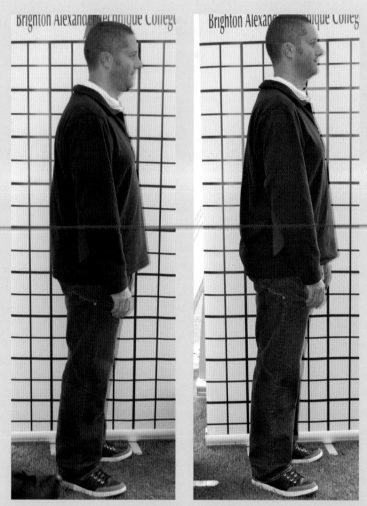

*These two photos, taken at a posture assessment stand in a health fair, show there is a clear difference between what you might consider poor posture and good posture. The photo on the left displays very clearly a man with a collapsed neck, which causes his head to jut forward. This in turn encourages his chest to be collapsed. His legs are stiff and his whole body is 'pulled down' towards the ground. You can describe this pattern as shortening in stature. His back is not lengthened, because of the pressures he puts on himself.*

*In the second photo, these issues have been resolved to a considerable degree. The man's neck is longer, more in harmony with his back, and his head is balanced well on the top of his neck. His whole body is 'longer' because the pulling down – which was an unrecognized over-activity of torso muscles – has been 'undone'. This man has not deliberately straightened up, but he has released tensions that were holding him down. In the second photo the man's posture is better than in the first, and the important thing is the way the man has set about getting there. Because he has achieved the changes by release rather than imposing yet another tension pattern on a collapsed structure, he is more likely to maintain the new way of supporting himself. It is effortless, and he was astonished at the difference not just in his outward appearance, but in the way he felt, which was lighter, freer and a revelation in balance.*

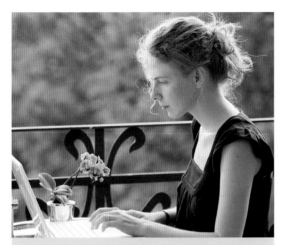

*If you work at your computer with your neck dropped like this it will complain – maybe not today, but in the end it will give you grief.*

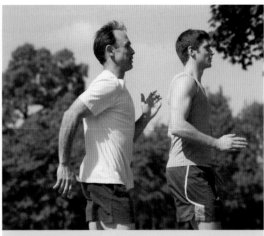

*Running with compression through your structure will damage you.*

more likely to injure yourself if you run with your neck tight and your head poked forward. But it won't be your neck you hurt – it will most likely be your back, which is being compressed from above by your stiff neck and head, and pounded from below by your heavy feet.

## Sort out your pain problems

Back pain is such a big problem that a lot of research has been done on how to cure or manage it. One significant clinical trial looked at the effectiveness of the Alexander Technique on low back pain and found that a course of 24 individual lessons reduced back pain considerably. People who reported 21 days per month in pain before lessons reported they had only three days per month in pain for up to a year after they had finished their lessons. They had learned to look after themselves better. Whereas it was once thought the best treatment for back pain was to avoid movement and lie flat on a board for days on end, it is now recognized that movement and exercise have a far better impact on morale, pain and mobility.

The question you have to consider is not just what exercise to carry out, but how to do it, how often, to what intensity and for how long at a time. Balancing rest and exercise is not easy, particularly if your pain makes you fearful that movement will set it off or make it worse. If you are concerned that your pain levels will increase with movement you are almost certain to hold your breath and interrupt its free flow. Attention to your posture and breathing is the first step to recovery, and best explored in active rest. Periods of active rest before and after exercise will greatly enhance your recovery. They will make you more accurate in your awareness of when to carry on a little longer and when to stop.

## Choose your activity

Only you know how severe your pain is, so only you can really decide how much to do, once you have all the facts. These guidelines assume you have had your problems checked out by your doctor and that you will use common sense! When it comes to exercising, consider hydrotherapy. Being in water and moving offers you support. It takes pressure off joints and lets you begin to tone up muscles that are out of condition.

I do not mean swimming, at least not straight away. There are specialist hydrotherapy pools

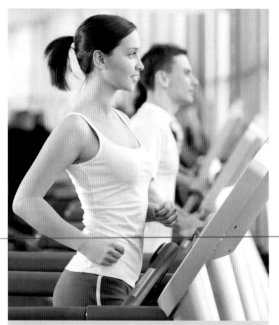

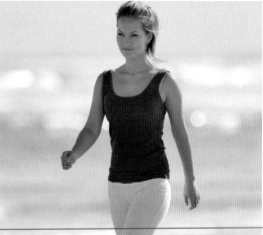

*Running with your back pulled in like this will not help your pain. It is more likely to transfer back problems to your neck. If you want to run, start with walking first and work on your thought–posture–movement. When you have that working well, start running a little at a time.*

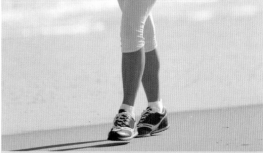

*Walking is an excellent way to improve fitness as well as help back pain. As with every exercise you undertake, you want to orientate your thoughts about your body upwards, so you constantly generate an upward impulse through your bones and muscles. It's always helpful to do some active rest before any exercise so that your directions are established.*

you can visit, or you can join an aquafit class. You might prefer to start by going to your pool when it is quiet and simply walking up and down in the water. Vary the way you walk, move backwards, forwards and sideways and notice how the water both supports you and makes demands on your muscles. Before you go to the pool, do some active rest so you start off with good coordination, and while you are walking, pay attention to your primary unity, and the sequence thought–posture–movement.

Start all your activities by directive thinking, 'I don't want to stiffen my neck'; followed by the posture consideration, 'I do want to free my neck and lengthen my back'; followed by the movement consideration, 'I'm walking through the water with my neck free and my back lengthening with my breath flowing'. You will find your active rest experience will help you keep this focus. Once

you feel happy with that, move on to rotational movements, still in water, drawing your arms across your body. This requires you to move the water against resistance, particularly if you use dumbbells as well. The key is always to stay with your thought–posture–movement sequence.

# Chapter 6
# Posture and breathing

**This chapter covers:**

- how we breathe
- specialized breathing
- breathing through the mouth and breathing through the nose
- sitting up straight
- signs of poor breathing

## How we breathe

As we breathe, so we are! Our breathing is largely dictated by our chosen postural norm. If that is a well-balanced one, breathing will be free and easy. If our norm is to hold ourselves with effort, or collapse and slump, then our breathing will reflect this. When considering ideas to help improve breathing, it's always good to remember that the Alexander Technique began with a man with a breathing problem, and at first he called his work 'respiratory re-education', and he would frequently say to people, 'allow the ribs to expand and contract'.

If your ribs have become immobilized, which can easily happen if your head and torso are being supported by clamping, your options for anything more than minimal breathing are very limited: you can either heave your whole rib cage up and down; or you can inhale with an excessive downward movement of your diaphragm, which in turn pushes your abdomen out and usually down, squashing your digestion as it does so.

Breathing is not something you can give up temporarily while you think about how to improve it. It's both an automatic activity, and one we can control. In other words, we don't have to think about it at all – we will continue to breathe even when asleep or not thinking about it. Our breathing will adapt to demand without our intervention – if we run our breathing will get deeper and quicker. If we relax on the sofa our breathing will be gentler and shallower.

We have the ability to control our breathing and this can work for us or against us because it is so easy for us to try and improve our breathing with no reference to our posture. If we do so – by doing deep breathing exercises or any breathing exercises – we don't help ourselves work with the important issue – what our breathing does when we are *not* thinking about it.

What are you doing when the breathing exercises are over? It is most likely that you resume your old, poor breathing habits, because without postural change there is no sustainable change in breathing behaviour. You breathe about seventeen times per minute (roughly speaking), which adds up to 25,000 breaths each day, quite a lot. So improving your breathing by properly understanding how it works is a worthwhile investment of your time and attention.

## Consider the diaphragm

The diaphragm is considered the main muscle of respiration because it is the one that moves the

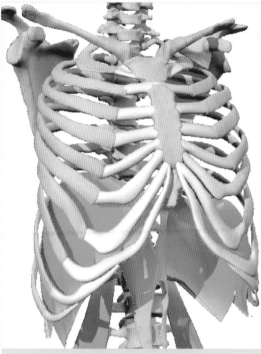 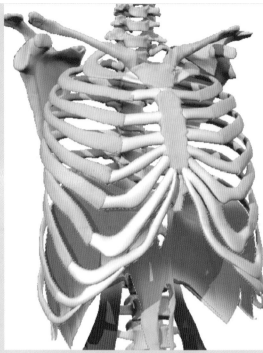

*The diaphragm, shown in green, is on an in-breath. It is toned as it descends downwards in the ribcage and the muscles that attach to the top rim of the pelvis are not very active either. This is the ideal scenario, and the framework of the ribcage is hardly disturbed at all.*

*The diaphragm on an out-breath is a little more relaxed and the back muscles are supportive as the diaphragm rises in the ribcage. If you are pulling your body down as you breathe, your respiration will be compromised.*

most when we breathe in and out. It makes room for our lungs to expand and take in air. It changes the internal pressures in our chest and abdominal areas and it is highly adaptive to demand. Other muscles of the back and torso are also important, because what they do – or don't do – crucially allows the diaphragm to move freely.

## Breathing in

Most descriptions of breathing concentrate on the action of the diaphragm as if it alone was responsible for breathing, and from a limited perspective this may be the case, but what you are doing with your entire body will influence your breathing directly. If you want your breathing to work freely and easily – and of course you do – then your body use must be such that it allows

your diaphragm the freedom to move as it needs.

So what does it do? When you take a breath in, your diaphragm flattens out from its dome-like shape and moves downwards. For many people this doesn't seem right because the ribs are lifting and it's easy to think the diaphragm is lifting too – but it isn't, it's descending. Your ribcage needs to make room for that to happen and should expand laterally. In other words, your ribs should flare outwards slightly and lift slightly too.

Your ribs have their own muscles to help you breathe, lovely little muscles that run diagonally up and down from rib to rib in both directions. There are three layers of them, the intercostals muscles, which are the ones you might injure if you develop a bad cough. As far as your ribs are concerned, coughing is exercise! If you cough vigorously you can make little tears in your muscles, as you will know if this has ever happened to you. If you are going to breathe well your ribcage needs to move both on your in-breath and your out-breath, and for that it needs support from your spine and torso.

In the two diagrams of the diaphragm, notice the muscle tails that are attached to the inside of the lumbar spine. Now imagine what the stress would be if you were very stiff and compressed in that part of your back. Those muscles would be compromised in their action. When you realize that those muscles blend in to the psoas muscles, which run down from the same place into the pelvis and on to the top of the legs, you can start to see why even tight legs just might make breathing more effortful.

## Breathing out

In quiet respiration, when you breathe out, your diaphragm is rising in your ribcage and your ribs are coming together, particularly the lower ribs, which should be flexible and move laterally towards your spine. This movement is often completely absent in the breathing cycle, and instead of lateral movement the whole rib cage is lifted up and dropped down again. This is hard work for your back and lungs.

# Poor breathing

If your habit of breathing is one in which every in-breath pushes your belly out and down, and every out-breath collapses your head, neck and thorax down into your belly, you will lack tone in the support musculature of your spine and belly, too. You may have tried to compensate for a flabby belly by holding it in. Sadly this won't help your breathe more easily – it will just tighten you up more. Poor posture invites distorted, restricted, shallow breathing and a host of other problems, including a ribcage that doesn't want to move, lowered vitality and poor concentration. Another common poor breathing pattern causes

your sternum (breast bone) to be sucked in so your whole chest looks collapsed and you will look either depressed or incredibly shy. In fact a shy person will tend to breathe differently from a confident one, and if the shy person learns to use their body better, and improve their posture and breathing, their confidence will rise. This is always accompanied by a rounded upper back, so trying to solve the problem by lifting your breast bone simply doesn't help. It always comes back to the same thing: your breathing is only as good as the scaffolding of your ribcage, spine and shoulder girdle, and the best way to improve your breathing is to improve your posture and body use.

## The subtle signs of poor breathing

If you are not lengthening it is likely that it's not just your back that slumps. If your knees or pelvis are locked, they block off energy flowing up and down your body, including through your spine. By 'energy' I mean blood flow, lymph flow and healthy muscle activity.

## Discover your breathing pattern

Try this little experiment to see how well your breathing and posture co-ordinate:

1. Stand easily on both legs for five natural effortless breaths, not too slow, not too fast.
2. Adjust your weight so you are standing more on one leg and count another five breaths.
3. Come back to centre and allow another five breaths to pass.
4. Shift onto the other leg and repeat.

Did you find it easier to breathe on one leg than the other? Which leg seemed to restrict your breathing most? Did you notice that when you are centred, breathing was easiest? The point is that even this seemingly insignificant 'posture' restricts your ease and depth of breathing, and eventually your energy. If you habitually stand slumped on one leg, you will restrict your breathing.

# Mouth or nose?

One significant fact which illustrates almost everything you need to know about your breathing is how you habitually breathe in. Is it through your mouth or nose? I'm talking about quiet respiration, rather than breathing while you are doing something demanding, such as singing or running. When you are at your computer and typing or sitting watching the television (on your supportive sofa of course!), how do you breathe? When you sleep does your mouth hang open so you breathe via your mouth and not your nose? If you are a habitual mouth breather you will fix your ribs – you almost can't avoid it. Think about a time when you had a heavy cold and a blocked nose – then you had to breathe through your mouth. If you did that all the time, you would help create problems for yourself.

## Filter hairs are in your nose, not your mouth

When you breathe through your nose, the air passes over your nose hairs, which help to filter out toxins and infections from the air. You don't want toxins in your lungs if you can avoid it. As the air travels to your lungs it is warmed up by the blood supply in your nose. This means the air hits your lungs at blood temperature, exactly what you want. Your lung tissue is delicate and reacts badly to very cold temperatures, which is why you automatically put a scarf over your mouth in very cold winter weather – you know you don't want that cold in your lungs.

Breathing through your nose is harder work physically than breathing through your mouth. It's very easy to prove that to yourself. Just try it out – take a big breath in through your open mouth –

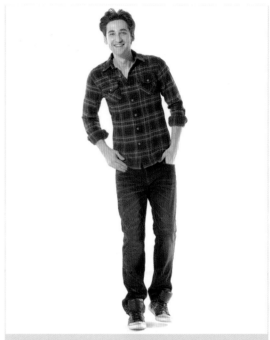

*Habitual leaning to one side affects breathing.*

easy isn't it? Now take a big breath in through your nose. Did it take longer to get the air in? Most likely (unless you are an athlete and a wizz at postural support and breathing).

There are other differences, too. When you breathe through your mouth your ribcage doesn't have to do much, so it gets lazy, stiff and what I describe as 'sullen', as if its own inertia gets more and more difficult to overcome and the work of respiration is passed to the abdominal muscles, which will do the job, but really need the support of a flexible ribcage to keep breathing easy.

If you breathe through your mouth habitually, you dry out the mucus linings in your throat, and fail to filter any toxins in the air. Your nostrils are the first line of defense when it comes to the air you breathe.

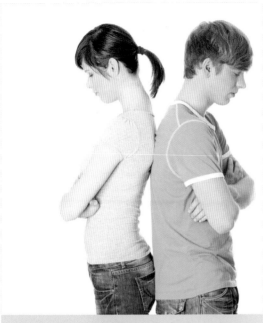

*Posture, breathing and attitude all influence each other. The two young people in the photo have restricted their breathing by their chosen posture of sulkiness. That's okay if it is quickly gone, but they both show poor posture, which is with them all the time. The woman's pulled in lower back and drooped neck speaks of many hours of poor posture, not just a teenage mood. The man's rounded shoulders tell the same story. It's not easy to maintain good postural habits if you constantly practice bad ones, so even when you are happy, you still have your bad habits, which show in walking, breathing and all your activities.*

## Experiment with posture and breath

Try this experiment to demonstrate to yourself how posture affects breathing. Sit down and bend forward as if you were going to tie your shoes, and now breathe in. Notice how much harder it is to breathe in when you are in this position. This is an extreme example of how your muscles and tendons can get over restricted and cause a lessening of depth and ease in breathing,

because of your bad posture. Of course you don't go around bent double all the time, but if you are slumping you will create the pressure you have just felt – to some extent at least. The pressures caused by bad posture also restrict your esophagus and vocal mechanisms, as well as breathing volume and ease.

## Sitting up straight

If you constantly have to remind yourself to sit up straight your body has adapted to be more comfortable in the slouching position. When you attempt to sit up 'straight', all you do is tighten the already over-shortened muscles down your front. This too interferes with ease of breathing volume; tightening these muscles even slightly to make yourself more erect causes tightness in your entire upper body and makes breathing even more difficult. This is usually enough to encourage you to slump again, because it was easier to breathe. That is why most people when advised to sit up straight only manage a few minutes of it before reverting to their former slouch, where breathing is a little easier. If this is your situation your breathing is not deep, easy and balanced. For you it has become easier to slump. But that can and should change!

### Case Study
#### Claire, mouth breather

Have you ever looked at your nostrils? Are they like little slits at the end of your nose, or are they wide and moving easily when you breathe? Do you breathe in and out through your nose or your mouth?

Standing Claire in front of my teaching mirror and asking these questions puzzled her a lot. She came for lessons because she'd heard it could help her asthma and she knew that her breathing

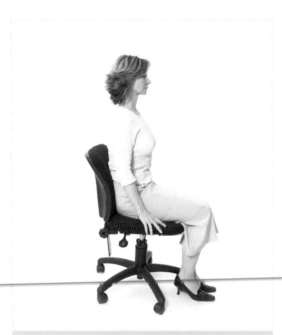

*Trying to force yourself to sit up straight will not last very long. Applying external muscular force to an internal organizational problem doesn't work.*

round her ribs and neck to help her appreciate the connection between her stiff tight neck and her fixed ribs, which was the result of years of poor breathing habits. As she began to let go of some of the tension in her neck, and keep her mouth closed as she breathed, her ribs started to creak back into life.

At first Claire felt a little panicky, concerned that she might not get enough air in through her nose, but we worked a lot with her lying in active rest and she soon found the panic diminish as her ribs moved and plenty of air came into her body. She learned to leave her shoulders alone, too, which had migrated right up round her ears because of her habit of sucking in air through her mouth.

After three months of lessons Claire met an old friend who said that Claire's neck had got longer and she looked taller. Claire told the friend she was having Alexander lessons and was learning to keep her mouth shut. 'About time too,' commented the friend.

was, as she put it, a bit poor. But she had no idea how important good breathing habits are and the effect poor breathing has on circulation and general wellbeing.

Claire's nostrils were indeed like little slits, which told me that she was largely a mouth breather. I pointed out to her that habitual mouth breathing makes your respiratory system lazy. It's much easier to take a breath in through your mouth than through your nose. Your ribs don't have to bother to move very much if you always breathe through your mouth. Your nose is lined with fine hairs to trap dirt and act as a filter, your mouth isn't! Your nose has a very good blood supply close to the surface, which makes the nasal lining warm so air is warmed to body temperature by the time it hits your lungs. Your mouth doesn't do that so in wintry weather very cold air hits your lungs and they don't like it. If you don't use your nose, it gets clogged up so stuffy sinuses are likely. This was Claire's situation. In our sessions I used my hands

# Breathing and speaking

If your breathing pattern is poor you might be holding your breath when you speak. This is common if you are in a tense situation where you feel stressed or nervous. If you do this, you are most likely to be pulling your body down as you speak, but still holding your breath. At the end of your sentence, or at other moments, you will let all your breath out in a rush and then gasp in another breath. This was F. M. Alexander's own breathing problem, which ultimately made him lose his voice when he was performing on the stage. He also realised that the poor breathing pattern was there when he wasn't speaking, too, and had profound effects on his stamina and general well being.

## Counting in a whisper

Although it is easy to hold your breath while you are speaking, it is almost impossible to hold your breath when you are whispering. Trying to do this is a way of becoming more aware of allowing your breath to flow more easily in speech. Try this experiment:

- Sit comfortably in balance on your sitting bones.
- Ask for your foundation lengthening up your back, and make sure your head is lightly balanced on the top of your spine.
- Make sure you keep the sense of lengthening through the breathing cycle.
- Take a breath in through your nose. It doesn't need to be an especially deep breath.
- Whisper from one to five. Make sure you don't voice the numbers, it must be a whisper. When you get to five, start at number one again.
- Count in cycles of one to five until your breath has almost run out.
- Don't try to force the counting.
- At the end of the counting, close your mouth and take in the next breath through your nose.
- Repeat the counting and taking in breaths three or four times and make sure you don't take any snatch breaths in between counts.

Gradually you will find your breathing settles into a gentle rhythm as you do this and you will be aware of your breath moving out of you as you whisper. You can then move on to counting out loud. This exercise will help you break the habit of holding your breath while speaking.

# Specialized breathing

The most useful way to work on your breathing is to consider what happens when you are not doing anything specialized. If you practice breathing for any meditation discipline or for playing an instrument, you will do so with the breathing patterns that are defined by your postural support. So the most useful way to think about breathing and to observe your own patterns is to practice active rest. This neutral exercise will reveal patterns or unnecessary tension that you may have developed unwittingly.

The two most common poor breathing patterns are either permanently raised shoulders, or such inflexibility in the ribs that the ribcage doesn't expand and contract freely. Both these patterns reveal themselves in active rest. For some people, the two patterns operate together and it can be a tangle to work out what is the best practice to unravel the tensions. This is where active rest can be so helpful. A free neck and a lengthening torso will allow breathing habits to reset themselves to a more harmonious pattern.

# Chapter 7
# Shoulder, arm, wrist and hand

## Most problems in hands, wrists and shoulders relate to the whole body

Our modern world is full of technology, much of which demands dexterity of hands and fingers. Many more people spend their entire working day at a computer, interspersed with texting or playing computer games. It's not uncommon for people to be doing more than one of these things at the same time. Quite apart from the sensory overload on your nervous system, there is a price to be paid for the excessive tension throughout your muscles, particularly through shoulders, arms, wrists and hands. If you have problems in these areas, you are faced with a tangle of issues to unpick. Most problems in hands, wrists and shoulders are either entirely created by, or reinforced by, over use or poor use not just of the part that is complaining, but of the whole body. The neck gets involved, the head is often dragged out of line by shoulder problems, and the whole back starts to accommodate to what is happening. In other words, your shoulder and wrist problem is likely to be a postural one.

## The shoulder girdle

Your shoulder girdle is made up of your two collar bones and your two shoulder blades, plus muscles and ligaments. Both these sets of bones are cleverly designed to give you maximum freedom for your arms and hands, which ultimately hang off your shoulder girdle. It's so mobile it's one of the easiest areas of your body to misuse. Your collar bones sit next to your breast bone and are connected to it by some grisly type tissue, but your shoulder blades float around in a sea of muscles on your back. They are not anchored by other bones, but lightly tethered with ligaments and muscles that mostly let them move around.

For you to reach up and comb your hair, your shoulder blades have to slide right over to one side of you. If you hold your hands together behind your back, they slide closer together. You can lift your shoulders up and down at will – it's part of your expression. The very mobility of your shoulder girdle lets you support it badly if you fall into bad habits. Your shoulder girdle does have its own supporting home – your ribcage, which allows the shoulders to 'sit' and move about freely. Your ribs in their turn are connected to your spine, and if your spine is collapsed then the support is lacking.

And so we come full circle again. What are you doing with your primary relationship of head, neck and back? If you lack harmony here, you will not have the proper support for your shoulders, arms and hands, which will then recruit your neck muscles to hold them up. Neck muscles are not really happy with this arrangement – they prefer to mobilize your head rather than stabilize your shoulders.

## Case Study
### Peter's frozen shoulder

Frozen shoulder is a very painful condition, affecting about 2% of the population, commonly in the 40–60 age group. Your shoulder becomes painful and stiffens up, and mobility is restricted. The pain can be so severe that everyday tasks such as combing your hair or getting dressed become very difficult. The cause of a frozen shoulder is not known, but it can last for up to two years. Although it is a very specific condition, it responds very well to a holistic postural approach.

When Peter rang me to say he'd been diagnosed with a frozen shoulder he was very fed up. His pain had come on gradually and he had ignored it until he couldn't tie his tie in the morning. He tried heat treatment and was taking anti-inflammatory drugs, which he disliked as they upset his stomach.

Peter's first surprise was discovering how much compensation he was doing throughout his body because his shoulder hurt. He was twisting his neck to one side, pulling the painful shoulder round, so his shoulder blade stuck out, and curling the fingers of his hand so tightly it was difficult

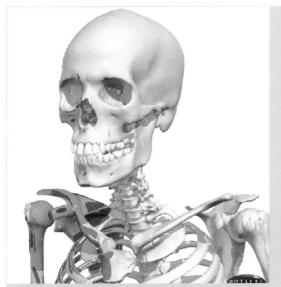

*Look how free and floating the bones of the shoulder girdle are. The coloured patches on the front view are where muscles and ligaments attach to the bones, letting you lift your arms and shoulders – otherwise how would you get your hat on – or take your jumper off? The back view shows some of the deeper muscle layers including those brave sub-occipital muscles at the base*

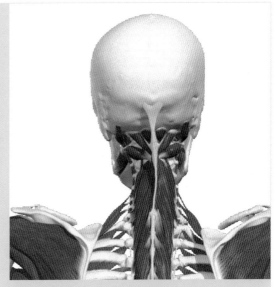

*of the skull – small but mighty! Notice how muscles chain down the back like a plaited rope; they are attaching your spine to your ribs, so if you persistently collapse your spine with terrible posture, these muscles have to shorten and tighten up – you leave them no choice.*

to straighten them. He adopted the active rest practice with extra support under his shoulder. He was surprised to be asked to think about his back and neck rather than his shoulder, but gradually he began to release the additional tension that had built up in his muscles. Even his legs were tense. Every bit of unnecessary tension makes it more difficult for a particular 'bit' of us to release fully. So learning to release your legs and back really does make a difference to shoulder problems.

After some time and practice, Peter said he felt calmer and noticed his breathing was easier. His shoulder was still stiff and painful but he felt he had learned something about how his whole body played a part in his tension. Pain levels decreased enough for him to be able gradually to stop taking his pain killers. He learned to notice when tension was building up in him and how to release it; his mobility improved and he was delighted with how much easier his breathing was.

Understanding how a part of you fits into the whole makes sense of why postural intelligence is so effective.

## Shoulder mobility; rotating the head of your upper arm bone

We spend most of our time working with our hands in front of us, and our shoulders rounded. This leads to a tightening of some of the muscles that flow off our chest and into the top of our arm. A big contributor to this shortened, round-shouldered posture is loss of rotational ability of the very top of our arm. The head of our upper arm, the humerus, has the ability to rotate in our shoulder socket, but it isn't a movement you tend to use during the course of the day, and perhaps because of this we easily lose that freedom, particular as we get older. But its loss encourages our whole shoulder, upper back and neck to become more fixed and rigid. Our shoulder blades tend to slide round and rise up instead of sitting relatively flat on our back. This in turn encourages

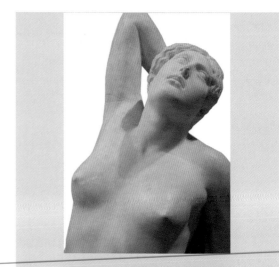

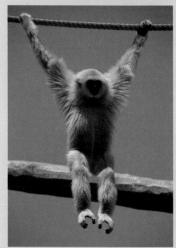

*The Greek statue and the monkey both demonstrate a wonderful rotation of the top of the arm in the shoulder socket. This enables your arm to be extended very easily over your head without compromising your neck, shoulders or head. So the monkey can use its arms with ease and swing from them freely and the statue can show us the possibility of that movement in a human. In both these examples the chest and shoulders are open, not hunched in any way. This rotation is almost a hidden movement, because you can put your arms over your head even if this rotation is only partial, but the result will be an uncomfortable narrowing of your chest and a lot of congestion in the shoulder and neck area – not the wonderful freedom of the statue or the monkey.*

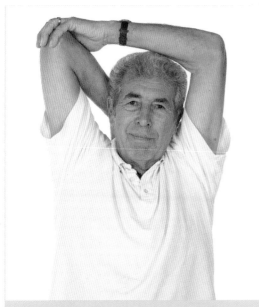

*Although this man has raised his arms successfully over his head, the lack of full rotation in his upper arm means his neck is compressed by the movement he has made. This compression has encouraged his neck to shorten and his upper chest to narrow as a result. With full rotation of the head of the humerus (the upper arm bone) he would get more benefit from this exercise.*

our ribcage, particularly the upper part, to become depressed and lose its mobility too. This fixation is unwittingly encouraged by sitting with rounded shoulders, particularly at a computer.

Rediscovering this movement can feel very strange and it may take you some time to 'find' the neurology to reconnect with this particular rotation. But when you do you will get a feeling of opening across your chest as well as a greater sense of freedom in your shoulder socket. For a full description of this and to try it out for yourself, *see* section 2 of the book, page 123–4.

# Specialist use of hands

In addition to what you might consider normal life – in which I include operating computers, phones and remote controls, chopping vegetables, and handling all the things you handle every day – there are specialist uses of the hands that make even greater demands on you. These include playing a musical instrument of any sort, activities such as knitting, and the use of small, delicate tools that require strength and precision – jewellery making is one such activity. Without sorting out your head, neck and back, your shoulders will be stiff, and when you then try and do something delicate or precise with your hands you are likely to bring in your neck muscles unnecessarily. Watch someone writing a cheque in a hurry and you will see they use their entire head, neck, jaw, shoulder and arm, just to do something their fingers should be doing. It's a huge waste of muscular energy.

## Playing an instrument

The higher your playing level, the greater the demand on your dexterity and strength. If you are playing at a professional level, you will already have learned a number of playing techniques and are likely to be practicing consistently every day over a long period of time, maybe years. Many dedicated musicians hone their skills and support their practice with the dedication of a top athlete.

One missing factor from specialist practice is often a sensitive postural and body use awareness, and this omission can be the downfall of a serious musician. If you have inadvertently created tension habits in your playing, you constantly re-enforce that tension to the point that you don't feel it possible to play without it. For some people this becomes an emotional security blanket. Familiar tension can appear comforting – purely because in the past it has enabled you to play. But the insidious advance of injury should tell you your playing technique really needs an overhaul. The overhaul is about you – not your specialized playing. It's about your postural intelligence, not your bowing or fingering technique. It's about the things you do when you are not playing.

# Trevelyan's story

Trevelyan Harper is a 20-year-old guitarist and drummer, a student on a modern music course, which involves him playing and practicing long hours. He is also tall and very lightly built, with a long neck and back. Although he suffered a lot of stiffness as well as pain, he has slightly lax ligaments. His structure is one that can be difficult to coordinate. Many tall, lightly built people experience back, neck or shoulder problems, particularly if they experienced a big growth spurt as teenagers. In the first year of his three-year course, Trevelyan ran into the kind of problems that can beset musicians, which not only result in pain and injury but also threaten studies and careers. Trevelyan had a series of Alexander lessons with me to address his use pattern and his postural problems. He agreed to keep a diary of his experience and insights. As his teacher, I have commented on elements of interest from a body-use point of view.

## My injury

My shoulder and neck injury began over a year ago, and seems to be the cause of the infrequent numbness in my thumb. My symptoms are numbness in the thumb with no physical pain. This seems to be brought about by using my thumb to either pincer or squeeze an object. This bothers me during guitar and bass playing, where I think the position of the wrist, combined with the force exerted when using my thumb as a pivot for the hand, brings on the numbness. When I have my guitar slung on a strap, or I'm carrying an excessive weight for some time on my left shoulder, the weight sets off the temperamental nature of the injury.

In the last two months this has subsided and the numbness is occasional; however, I still have a tight and aching neck and shoulder and sometimes back. For a long time I have been sure this is related to posture and imbalance.

# Carolyn's comments

*I was most interested in Trevelyan's early experience of numbness with no pain, and his observation that this might have been brought about by a particular pincer action of his thumbs – action he needs in order to play. This already suggests to me the problem is largely influenced by his primary control – the coordination of his neck, head and back. With a long neck and back, and his light build, his whole structure makes it more difficult for his shoulder girdle to 'sit' on his ribcage and get the right support from his back and ribs. Usually this support is then recruited from elsewhere in the body – often the neck, which isn't designed for it. All his observations, which were very accurate, go to support this idea.*

## Diagnosis and treatment

After a few futile weeks of rest I sought help from a physiotherapist in Brighton who was recommended to me by one of my course tutors. After a few sessions she identified the problem as an injury to my shoulder, neck and second rib. This area seemed to be the cause of the problems in my hand. The treatment involved massage to the shoulder and surrounding area, which did barely anything. The physiotherapist wrote a letter to my doctor, who administered a steroid injection into my shoulder. This was in July, nearly four months after the injury started. For the first seven weeks or so of the summer this seemed to 'cure' the injury, but in reality I think it just numbed the area affected and the drug inevitably wore off.

I went back to the physiotherapist clinic and saw a different physiotherapist, who administered similar massage treatment to no avail. I had a session one week with a physiotherapist who revealed to me that none of the treatment I was being given was actually intended to cure the problem. It was merely designed to alleviate the symptoms of my injury. This disheartened me somewhat, and I stopped seeing the therapists.

In the meantime I had been trawling through the slow NHS system seeing professionals. I had a brief session with a specialist in the rheumatology department in Eastbourne, who sent me to have an MRI scan. The results came back showing nothing. He then sent me to see someone in the neurological department, who tested my nerves with electrodes and other things, but this revealed my nerves aren't damaged. I am now on the waiting list to see another specialist at the hospital next month. When I was offered the chance to have some Alexander Technique lessons I decided to try it.

## Carolyn's comments

*Trevelyan's experiences re-enforced for me the fact that it was his basic pattern of use that was the problem. Rest is always helpful, but if you then start doing things the way you always have done them, the problem will return. It is always difficult to get back to the real influence on an injury – and this was precisely Alexander's own journey. He discovered the nature of his primary control of his entire body, and how to influence it for positive support. This is going to be Trevelyan's journey too.*

## My first lesson

I went along to my first session knowing little if anything about the Alexander Technique. Other than the fact it is related to posture and correct movement of the body, I had no preconceptions of what the technique entails. As I now understand it, it is the process of releasing the muscles in the body and synchronizing them to work together when making a movement, instead of pulling against each other in opposite directions as they do through bad habit.

The process of doing this seems to me to take the body through common movements or positions, such as standing up and sitting down, standing still and lying down. With the guidance of my teacher, who uses her hands on me to facilitate these movements, it seems not only to correct the posture, but also to remind the body and mind what it is like when the muscles are relaxed and working together. Once the body knows what this

feels like, the neural pathways will automatically be telling the muscles to release and it will become a good habit as easily as it became a bad habit.

It seems we have connections to our body and our muscles beyond our immediate conscious commands. This is why the technique of 'telling' your muscles to release with your mind, rather than directly relaxing them, has an impact on how we conduct ourselves in a given position or movement.

## Carolyn's comments

*Spot on! Musicians are usually highly sensitive to their bodies, and when offered a fruitful way of working with themselves, they respond well. Trevelyan's first lesson gave him tools to work with straight away, such as active rest, where he could build the skills of good body use and improve his awareness of what he was actually doing habitually, as opposed to what he believed he was doing. This is a difficult lesson, because we are often deeply wedded to our feelings of what is 'right' in our bodies, and it takes an open mind to challenge that belief. Trevelyan has the right kind of curiosity to let him experiment.*

## Trevelyan's Alexander journal

### Thursday 4 Feb

I spent twenty minutes lying down as instructed today. Interestingly I felt remarkably comfortable, and as instructed I attempted to send 'commands' to my neck to release. I did this for a short while, and then my mind began to wander. When I focused on it again, I seemed to feel a change, a change far more prominent and noticeable than my initial trial of this exercise. It was a most strange sensation where my neck almost felt like it was moving or adjusting itself in a subtle manner, seemingly without direct instruction or prompt. The change was small but still noticeable.

After this feeling my neck seemed more comfortable and relaxed and I spent the rest of the time 'instructing' my tailbone to reach towards the door and my neck to reach towards the window, which is situated in the opposite direction. However, this did not yield any noticeable results.

### Friday 5 Feb
I spent twenty minutes again today lying down. I experienced similar results to yesterday. The feeling of release in my neck seemed to last longer this time.

### Friday 12 Feb
It has been a week since my last entry. Although I have only managed to take the time to practice the exercise three times this week, it has yielded good results. I have also spent this week focusing on releasing my muscles in my neck whenever I come to think of it, which seems to be more and more often.

## Carolyn's comments
*Trevelyan's experiments directing his lying semi-supine (in active rest) are starting to improve his awareness. His observation that he seems to think of releasing his neck more frequently is particularly interesting, because this is how it works. The time spent in active rest, where you are paying a lot of attention to yourself and what is going on in your neck and back, increases your awareness when you are up and about your daily life. Every time Trevelyan thinks of releasing his neck, he makes it more sensitive to misuse and easier to release. He is literally teaching his muscles a different way of supporting his head.*

## Trevelyan's Alexander journal
### Thursday 18 Feb
This week has been similar to last week. I am eager to have my next session as I strongly feel I would benefit from knowing how to correctly practice doing chores and other activities with correct posture. I notice that when I'm drumming and doing simple activities like washing up, there is strain in my neck. Drumming can make my shoulders and neck very stiff and tight, and a

prolonged time doing this activity will leave an aching feeling.

### Saturday 20 Feb
I spent 25 minutes lying down today, as instructed. I experienced a similar release of the neck. I am curious to know if I'm sleeping correctly. Some mornings I wake up and my hand feels fine, I can play normally. Other days I wake up and my shoulder is aching. This impedes my guitar playing.

### Monday 22 Feb
At band practice today I realized that my shoulder has significantly improved. Three hours of standing up with the guitar slung across my shoulder used to be too much for it, and I would start getting numbness, but this has improved significantly. I am also curious to know how to sit correctly at my computer as prolonged sessions leave my neck and shoulder feeling achy.

## Carolyn's comments
*The primary control is something that is there all the time. You can use it well – or badly. If you don't know about it – or you ignore it – your habits just take over and they may not serve you well. It doesn't matter what you're doing – the washing up, sitting at the computer, or playing the guitar. Trevelyan has realized this, and is aware too that even good use of the body requires you to be intelligent about how long you engage in demanding activities.*

## Trevelyan's Alexander journal
### 15–23 March
This past week has shown the most substantial evidence so far for the benefits of the Alexander Technique with regards to my injury. I feel it has been the most productive week in the application of the technique and its concepts.

I have worked on the concept of inhibition and applying it to both my playing and my everyday life. I believe I have made several steps in the right direction, for example, inhibiting the muscles that habitually tense themselves whenever I go to play the guitar. This has been particularly effective when I have spent 20 to 30 minutes lying down in 'active rest' and concentrating on lengthening and releasing my neck. I then move straight to the guitar and try to keep that same release of the muscles. This is something that is actually quite difficult, but I believe I am coming closer to doing it effectively. I have also tried applying this to playing drums although to a lesser extent.

Having spent much time at the computer throughout the last week or so I have given extra consideration to my posture and release of my neck while typing or playing games. I have found that frequent 'active rest' breaks from any activity throughout the day have been most beneficial in dispelling any residue of tension that has built up. This also serves to remind my body frequently of the correct posture and release.

One of the most pleasing changes of late is that I can play acoustic guitar again! For a long period of time after my injury I couldn't play the acoustic guitar because the added string tension, thickness of the neck and action of the guitar meant it required more force from my thumb, thus bringing on the dreaded numbness. After returning home at the weekend I found I could play the acoustic guitar and have been gradually playing more and more every day since, slowly easing myself back into it. This is a change I am attributing to the Alexander Technique as I have found an irrefutable connection between how good my posture is and how temperamental my injury is being.

## Carolyn's comments

*When someone grasps the concepts of inhibition and direction, it really is like finding the keys to the treasure box! Taking frequent active rest breaks is an excellent way of dispelling tension and resetting good habits. It's so nice to have a thoughtful student!*

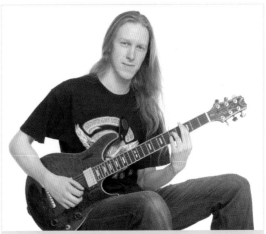

*This is Trevelyan demonstrating excellent use of his head and neck. He is able to do what he needs to do in order to play without causing himself pain.*

## Trevelyan's Alexander journal

### My progress with the Alexander Technique

The last few weeks have been very productive as I have practiced and applied the Alexander Technique. Much of my active rest practice has been geared towards gaining release in the shoulders and chest area as I seem quite able to release my neck at will now.

I have found that during activities such as walking, running, swimming, standing up, sitting down, drumming and guitar playing I have been able to carry out the actions with a good amount of release in my neck and back. Obviously this is an ongoing practice and I have far more release to be gained while doing these activities, but the results of the application of the Alexander Technique are there and I can feel it!

Following a recent reprise of my injury due to over playing I have had to cut down on practicing. However, this forced my mind to focus more on the application and practice of the Alexander Technique so some good came of this relapse.

Over the last two weeks, when I have done little or no playing at all, I have had more time and ultimately more need to practice releasing my shoulder to help the injury heal, which it has done successfully. I am now back playing and practicing, edging my way back up to my previous level of practice.

Another application of the Alexander Technique that I have focused on recently is my posture and release while at the computer. Because I have had many assignments and essays over the last few weeks I have spent many long sessions at the computer. After the first few long sessions I was left with an achy back so I reassessed my set up, raised the monitor on top of a pile of books and focused on typing with a released neck. I used the technique looked at in one of my sessions to gauge how released my neck was. It involved using one hand to feel the palm of my other hand while it was typing, and seeing if there was unnecessary tension in it (see the exercise in the section 'How tense are your hands?' opposite). I found this helped greatly and I could sit comfortably at the computer for far longer and could focus more because I wasn't distracted by tension in my back and neck.

I have recently started reading F. M. Alexander's book **The Use of the Self** and have found that my understanding of the technique is growing. I found the idea about sensory untrustworthiness very fascinating and very true to me. Throughout much of my study of the technique I have experienced the difficulty in actually knowing whether what I'm doing is right or wrong. It is very hard to stop trusting one's senses in the way you always have and to trust them in a different way. It takes a while to actually become aware of the tension in oneself, but this has to be mastered before one can begin releasing this tension.

I am still reading the book and I'm finding it very interesting. I hope to gain a new level of understanding about the technique once I finish it.

## Carolyn's comments

*Trevelyan completely self-manages his situation now. He uses active rest intelligently, and his awareness of his own interference patterns is excellent, as is his willingness to approach them differently. I'm very impressed that he is reading Alexander's* The Use of the Self. *This contains a description of Alexander's experiments with his posture and use, and records many blind alleys and 'back to the drawing board' moments. In*

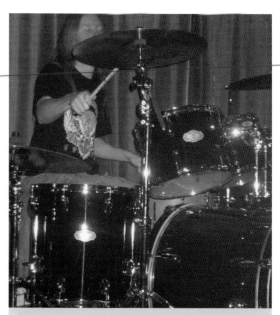

Drummers notoriously suffer neck, back, shoulder and wrist problems. Good organization of your back and neck gives support to your shoulders and arms.

*particular the area of unreliable sensory awareness is well documented by Alexander and reflects Trevelyan's experience.*

## Trevelyan, two years on

Yesterday I arrived in Santiago. I have been walking across Spain for the past fifteen days. We've done around 380km with full back pack load. The Alexander Technique has been very helpful. I've been doing my semi-supine practice after every journey and it has really helped out!

## How tense are your hands? Try Trevelyan's experiment

Practicing this exercise is a good way to recognize tension in your hands. You can adapt it to all sorts of situations to get an idea of what your hand is up to when active. First of all try this sitting at a table – the kitchen table will do nicely.

Start with one hand in a loose cup shape, as if you were holding a tennis ball, palm up. Then turn it over and rest your fingertips on the table, still keeping the cup shape. This is your active hand. Very gently place the tips of one or two fingers of your other hand (your enquiring hand) in your palm, from the bottom, so you can feel the underside of the palm of your active hand. You might need to organize your hands a bit so you are comfortable doing this, perhaps bringing them both more towards your midline so it's easy. If it helps, lift your thumb off the table, so your enquiring hand has easy access to your palm. The fingertips of your enquiring hand are now in contact with the tendons that supply the fingers of your active hand, so tap those fingers up and down and see what you can feel.

If those tendons feel like little ropes, not only is your hand tense, your whole arm, shoulder and neck are tense. So start in the right place – your neck – and ask that to release before you release the hand. You will notice a big difference. You need only a little tendon activity to operate your hand – nothing like as much as you usually have.

If you play the piano or any other keyboard, you can transfer your experiment to the keyboard and try playing little patterns, such as you might do in learning scales. You will soon find you need far less tension than you thought. Replace tension with direction and you will get dramatic results. The other place to try this out is at your computer. It's the same idea. Get your hands set up so one fingertip is monitoring your palm and type away. Always remember the role your neck plays in all this and experiment until you can type with almost no tension in your hands.

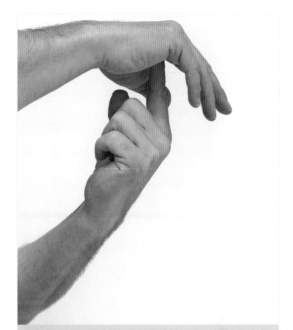

*When you monitor an active hand, the first thing to try is simply to wiggle your fingers in this position. Having tuned in to your hand tendons, you can adjust your hands to any situation you want, like typing or playing the piano.*

## The terrible tight thumb

Your thumb is at the end of a pattern of spiralling muscles that run round your arm, up into your chest and shoulder, and attach at the front and back of your skull. If your shoulder girdle lacks support, this spiral will shorten through its length, not only dragging your shoulders up to your ears, but also making your thumb stiff. This will effectively jam your wrists up, too. This can happen as a result of too much time spent in activities that encourage shortening. Early signs are an inability of the hand to lie flat on a table easily.

Of course you can flatten it with effort, but don't do that. Lie your hand and forearm on a table and have a look at it. Casually lay your hand palm down

87

on a flat surface; what does it look like? Because our thumbs can be overactive, all the muscles of the thumb and forearm shorten and drag the thumb into the wrist. This shows itself as a tight arch at the base of the thumb. The index finger is also dragged out of shape by a tight thumb and tends to 'lift' as it is pulled inwards towards the palm. At its worst, the whole hand becomes tense, narrowed and claw like. The hand in the photo below shows the first signs of poor use.

If your hand exhibits these tendencies it's time to do something about it. Section 2 contains several exercises to help you undo the bad habits that got you shortening. If your hands are your livelihood, either because you play an instrument or you are a masseur, you need to look after them in the context of your whole posture.

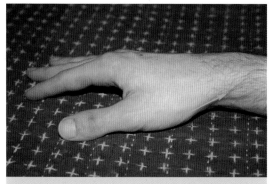

*The green arrows indicate the direction of pull of the thumb into the wrist, and the shortening of the index finger side of the hand. This can lead to the wrist becoming stiff and inflamed. The muscles of the forearm help drag the thumb inwards. Reversing this takes time but is very effective in relieving pain and tension.*

# Chapter 8
# Posture in performance

## The foundation of activity

Posture plays many roles in our lives. It makes up our fundamental relationship with gravity and is with us all the time. There is nothing we do that doesn't involve our posture in some way. As well as being important for our health and wellbeing, posture is a key consideration in all types of performance, as the way we use our bodies either helps or hinders us. When we engage in any form of specialist training, it is all too easy to overlook this most useful tool – our coordination and how we create support in our bodies in order to move. There is little point in training intensively to learn to play tennis or the piano if you can't manage your postural support first and foremost.

## Sports

We all want to keep fit, and are encouraged to take part in sports to improve flexibility, strength and help with weight management. But sports can lead to injuries, and some of these are due to poor coordination rather than other risk factors.

F. M. Alexander highlighted the importance of what he called the primary control. This is the all-important relationship you have between your head, neck and back. This relationship determines the way you cope with gravity. So if you constantly stiffen your neck and retract your head, and then decide to take up tennis, you are more likely to injure your neck and shoulder than if you have good coordination and your basic posture isn't already causing you stress.

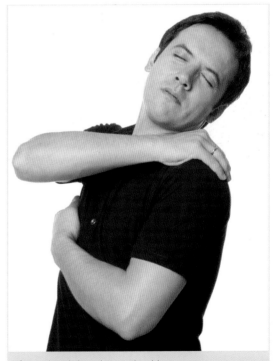

*If you already hunch your shoulders you are more likely to have problems if you take up tennis, which demands both strength and flexibility in the shoulders.*

# Singing and acting

Actors and singers also pay a lot of attention to their posture. Many of them practice long hours and suffer from injuries caused by stress, often related to poor posture and poor coordination. When the stakes are high, good posture is essential and something that has to be thought about all the time. I asked international opera singer Neil Jenkins to outline some of the challenges he has dealt with in his long singing career. Some of Neil's stories are hair raising – singing a battle cry standing on the end of a narrow plank jutting out over a long drop with no safety net is not usually what one thinks of when deciding on an operatic career, but it was all in a day's work for Neil.

Neil Jenkins has been a professional singer for over forty years. He is equally at home as an operatic, oratorio or recital singer; and combines this with work as a musicologist. Neil has sung with all of Britain's opera companies, especially Kent Opera, Scottish Opera and Welsh National Opera, and at Glyndebourne. Opera singing is an athletic activity, which makes enormous physical and emotional demands on a singer's body. Throughout his career, which now includes teaching and conducting, Neil has been a keen student of the Alexander Technique, which has helped him cope with the stresses and strains of his profession and to recover from injuries. Neil agreed to talk about the importance of posture and reveal some of the conditions he has coped with.

# A raked stage

For an audience to have a good view of performers on all parts of the stage, the stage is often raked so it is higher at the back than the front – it's a slope. The higher the rake the better the audience's view, but the more difficult it is for the performers who have to cope with it. They may have an upstage entrance and have to walk down stage – downhill. If the stage is shiny or slippery in any way it can cause considerable problems. Walking on a raked stage requires adjustment in balance and, according to Neil, plays havoc with the backs of your legs. You have to compensate all the time, through your legs, buttocks and back. If you turn sideways on to the audience, your upstage leg is more bent than your downstage one and you have to compensate for that as you walk across stage. Your walk must look natural, not as if you are walking sideways across a hill, which is in fact what you are doing. When you face straight forward your ankles are slightly extended and your feet tipped away from you, so you grip in the backs of your legs to hold yourself in position.

# Female roles in heels

As a high tenor, Neil was much in demand for female roles. He had to wear high heels and learn to walk in them on a raked stage, avoiding complicated bits of scenery, walking up and down steps and generally moving about the stage. Playing female roles often involves wearing a corset, as well as additional padding. Not only did Neil have to learn how to manage all of these obstacles, but he had to sing, too – and sing well. So he had to find a way to produce his voice under these difficult conditions, and make it look easy and natural, so the audience was completely unaware of any stresses and strains and saw only a lively, animated performance with top quality singing. He commented:

*High tenor rules are great fun to sing, but learning to walk comfortably and naturally in high heels is quite an art, and being on a raked stage in a complicated set put extra strain on me where there wasn't strain before. I think that's where my back problems started. Despite all these physical problems you have to sing the roles, which are demanding and high, so you have to position the voice in a particular way and that is mostly what you are thinking about. So tensions come along and pain creeps in.*

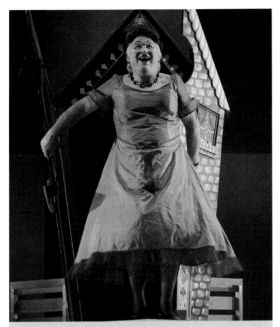

*Neil as the Witch in* Hansel & Gretel *(Welsh National Opera). Coping with heels, padding and the weight of a costume can put strain on the performer's back.*

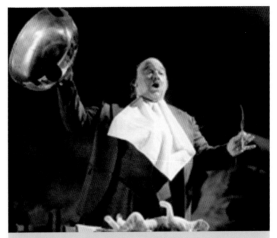

*Neil as Irus in* Return of Ulysses *(Welsh National Opera)*

# Wearing the costume

When we see a performance, we see the performers in their costumes only on the stage and have no idea how long they might have to wear them at other times. When a performance is in rehearsal, coming up towards opening night, all the elements are drawn together – the staging, the orchestra, the lighting, the sound. Everything has to be balanced and work together, and this takes time. A singer might spend up to nine hours in rehearsal, much of it waiting while other things happen, and most of that time in costume. The more complicated the costume, the longer it takes to get into and the more reluctant dressers are to let singers take it off. Some costumes are so complex that a singer has to be dressed by someone else (a dresser) and couldn't take it off unaided anyway. Neil recalls one role in particular:

*I recently played the role of Irus – a glutton – in Return of Ulysses. For this I wore a fat suit under the main costume. Fat suits are difficult to get into; it's such a palaver that once in it you don't take it off just for a short break, or lunch. It's very hot; you sweat buckets, especially when you are under the stage lights. On top of the fat suit I wore another three-piece suit, which was also hot. It's your shoulders that take all the punishment, carrying the weight of the costume.*

# Favorite costumes

Neil enjoys wearing eighteenth-century costumes, as he feels they help you stand elegantly. Your posture is very upright and your arms are not held tightly against your body, so as a singer you have so much more freedom for your ribs to expand than in some other costumes where you still have to expand your ribcage to sing, but it can be a struggle. Even wearing what he describes as glorious robes, which can be very heavy and a weight on the shoulders, doesn't daunt him:

*You need your shoulders to stay down, to stay low, for singing opera, so robes are wonderful for that. But it is a relief to take them off.*

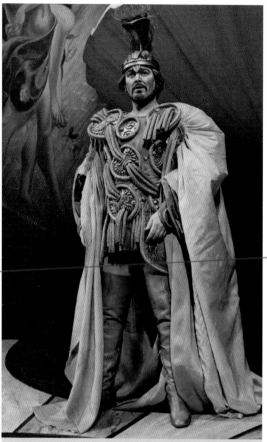

*'Glorious robes', as Neil calls them, can be so heavy that a singer needs help to put them on and take them off. Notice the well-balanced stance, with wide spaced legs and open shoulders Neil has adopted in this role. It enables him to take the breath he needs for singing. With a heavy helmet to balance on his head, he has to ensure it looks good too, while still keeping enough space in his neck to sing.*

## Double costumes

Singers may take two roles in an opera and usually there is time to change costume from one role to the other, but sometimes this is not possible and another solution has to be found. A director is focusing on the effect he or she wants to create

and the singer has to work to the guidelines offered. Neil reflected on how tricky it is to work in some costumes:

*Sometimes costumes can just be very awkward and uncomfortable. I was in a performance of The Magic Flute [by Mozart] at Glyndebourne – a Peter Sellars' production – and I was playing the role of Monastatos, a nasty creature really, and I had a purple face, very heavy make up. I was also doubling up as an armed man and for this I had to wear a decontamination suit and a helmet to cover my purple face. There was no time in between coming off stage as Monastatos and going on as the armed man for me to change costume, so I had to put the decontamination suit on over the suit I was already wearing and then the helmet. It was extremely hot and restrictive. Despite drinking a lot I ended up in hospital with kidney stones, and really it was due to wearing that double costume. You don't think about it like that – it's just your job and you get on with it. Your body has to get into all sorts of strange shapes and positions, and each role is different.*

## Dealing with scenery

If the costumes don't get you the scenery will. Opera is a spectacle and scenery is a big part of it. Stages are not static; scenery can move quite dramatically. This too can be challenging. Neil recalls a particular performance in Lyon where he was playing Oberon in a performance of Weber's opera of the same name, and the stage designer and director wanted a clever set that moved significantly:

*The floor of the stage was on a hydraulic lift and could move through 90 degrees so that it became a wall. I was lying asleep on the floor, draped over a rock, not a very comfortable position. I was covered with a sheet. Puck came in, flying above me on a wire, as the music played and the floor started to move, changing slowly from horizontal to vertical. I would eventually end up upright about nine feet off the ground.*

*The movement made me feel quite dizzy because my body would still be moving when the stage stopped. So I needed to be very secure and was attached to the wall with a pair of seat belts. This meant I couldn't fall off the wall. I also had a small platform underneath my feet to stand on when I became upright. It really was very small, not much bigger than an A4 sheet of paper, so I was secured to the wall with two quick release belts, one round my upper chest, just under my arms, and another round my hips.*

*All went well until the dress rehearsal, when the platform under my feet gave way just as I got upright and I was left dangling, like a crucified Christ supported only by the belts, which were getting tighter and tighter. I yelled out in French – 'I'm falling, I'm falling can you bring down the curtain!' – and the audience, believing it was part of the performance, laughed uproariously. It took quite a while for the stage manager to realize that something had gone disastrously wrong and to bring the curtain down.*

*I broke a rib doing that. But the show was opening the next day and so I had to carry on and sing twelve performances with a broken rib, which was agony to sing with, because of course as you're expanding your lungs, so the lungs are pressing on the rib. After that I checked the bolts on the platform personally before every performance! So one puts one's body through a lot of punishment because sometimes things go wrong.*

## Concerts

After the terrors of costumes, stages that disappear under your feet and helmets that choke you, you might think that concert work is a safer option. At least you won't be in danger from your clothes, or practically strangled by scenery and props. Neil's dress shirts are always two collar sizes larger

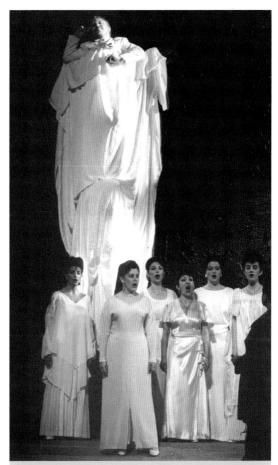

Neil (as Oberon) has to stand on this tiny platform for over twenty minutes, and sing an aria and a duet with Puck.

than his actual size so there is plenty of room for his Adam's apple to move up and down freely. Concerts have different challenges and different obstacles to maneuver around, not least an orchestra. So there is still the question of space around you and your balance within the space.

Neil remembered the first time he sang at the Royal Albert Hall:

*I got vertigo. In between rehearsal and performance the conductor had rearranged everything. There was an orchestral piece first before me, and of course I hadn't rehearsed with that, but it meant*

93

*that when I walked out to do my bit, live of course, there were more players on the stage than when I'd rehearsed my part earlier. So there was only a tiny place at the edge of the stage for me to stand. My toes were literally at the edge of the stage and I felt I could easily fall off.*

*As my career advanced I got pernickety about this and insisted on a better arrangement. One of my favorite works is the Britten* Serenade for Tenor, Horn and Strings *and I want to be as far back as possible from the edge of the stage so I'm amongst the musicians and I have room to breathe and expand. I would normally stand on the side of the orchestra [by] the 'cellos. So I insist that the 'cellos are pushed back a bit. It's all a question of balance. You can't sing if you feel that everything is too close around you. If you can't get your balance properly you can't do your best.*

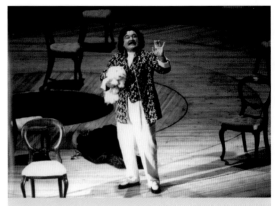

*Neil taking his weight onto his back leg to support his voice production.*

# Good posture for singing

Over the course of a long career of singing and teaching Neil has had ample opportunity to see the common errors singers make in their posture and how this affects their performance. In particular the temptation to pull forwards. In Alexander terms we sometimes refer to this phenomenon as 'losing the back', meaning that you have disengaged from the support your back should offer you. This habit is common in people seeking to communicate in any way, acting, singing or public speaking. When the back is not properly engaged you lose postural and vocal support; you almost literally take the stuffing out of yourself and have nothing to place your voice on. Neil describes what happens when singers want to communicate:

*One of the things I feel singers want is to communicate, and they often lean too far forward, because they think that somehow by doing so* they're reaching the audience better. The more I have been at this business, and also taught, which helps one see what should be happening, the more I see that really one wants to be back. You want to be balanced on a leg that's behind you. It's almost like you want to make a tripod, but of course you've only got two legs to work on – so you have an imaginary leg behind you, so you get strength coming up it and into the back. That is the way you can feel more comfortable in an awkward situation.*

# Experiment with Neil's 'tripod' leg

As you walk and take weight over your legs, they tone up to support you. That tone connects right through your back, and this is what Neil is cleverly making use of. To experience this yourself, try the following:

- Stand with your feet side by side, but with a small gap between them. Stand easily, with your knees straight but not locked, your neck free from tension and your head and back directing upwards.
- Take a small step backwards with one foot and slowly bring your weight over it

so you are standing more on the back leg than the front one.

■ Notice that this action encourages tone throughout your whole back. This tone not only supports you physically, but gives you strength so you feel comfortable in an awkward situation

You can recreate that support in your back with your feet side by side, by mentally stepping back onto one leg, or imagining a tripod third leg behind you, as Neil sometimes does. This directed thought creates a physical change in your body and your back works better.

# More about legs

F. M. Alexander was an actor and reciter; in particular he excelled at reciting long narrative ballads, which have a rhythmic form and character similar to singing. Both demand superb breath control and awareness. Like singing, they are spoken on an exhalation, when air is going out, not when it is going in. To be sure that the air (on which you either speak or sing) is going out of you easily and in the way you need to fuel your voice, the in-breath needs to be effortless too. This is only possible when posture and body use are well organized; if legs are tense or badly used, they interfere with posture rather than supporting it.

When he was a young man, one of F. M. Alexander's drama teachers told him to 'take hold of the floor with your feet'. He interpreted this by unwittingly tensing his legs and in so doing he disturbed the muscles of his back, making them rigid and inflexible. This in turn made it difficult for his ribs to move well, so his breathing was compromised and his speaking voice adversely affected, causing him to become hoarse very easily. In the course of discovering good body use and drawing together the element that became the Alexander Technique, he completely rethought his interpretation of this strange instruction

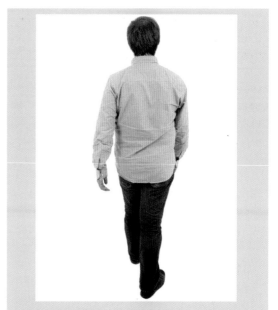

*Take time over this apparently simple activity. Make sure you don't lean heavily on the supporting leg; instead, think 'up' off it so you allow your body's natural spring to work.*

'take hold of the floor with your feet', until he understood, and ultimately taught, that a free neck allows for a lengthened back and legs. This length is not mere relaxation: it is elastic strength that brings the feet into a firm but springy contact with the floor. This is what Neil does as a singer. He creates a good contact with the floor by a sensitive and thoughtful use of his legs and feet.

## Owning the space

The size of the venue a singer performs in makes different demands. It's not just a question of acoustics, although that is important. The singer must understand the space so he or she can inhabit it properly. Singers and actors have to cultivate this skill to a high degree. It is what makes us, the audience, able to engage fully in the performance, even to believe we are somewhere we are not. We can be made to believe we are in a cherry orchard, whereas in fact we are in a run-down vacant shop. The ability to transform space is largely achieved through the singer's or actor's posture and body awareness. This ability to occupy space is crucial for Neil, who might find himself singing in venues ranging from a small barn to a cathedral, the Royal Albert Hall, an opera house or someone's front room.

Neil describes how he achieves it, using his placement within the space to reflect back into his posture and awareness:

*I was doing live television, a performance of Britten's Serenade, which is probably one of the hardest things that I do, and it was being filmed in Worcester Cathedral. In order to help me get my focus right, and my thoughts, I would go and sit in the building for a while and get to know the building so it felt friendly, and felt like my building rather than being a very strange environment. So I knew I had to go in – and there's this building – and over there [Neil conjures up an imaginary pillar with his hands] is a pillar that I knew I would want to look at, that was a friendly pillar. I knew I could make that pillar friendly, and it would give me strength. That's how I would get to a situation where I could be that strong [to sing well].*

By relating to a pillar, Neil orientated his posture and position in space. He could move around freely, knowing the position of the pillar won't change. This enabled him always to know exactly where he was and the resulting confidence allowed him freedom of body and mind, a vital condition for singing.

## Dealing with nerves

When you perform in a large public place, at famous events and famous venues, it can be very intimidating. The Royal Albert Hall can seat over 8,000 people and is home to the world famous Proms. Neil describes how he adapted his posture and mental attitude to cope with the challenge of singing at the Proms:

*One of the terrifying things for me was to walk out onto the stage of the Royal Albert Hall and do a live prom. People said to me 'I don't know how you can do that', and I said, 'Well, I just lift my chest, and get my balance right [over my feet] and walk out with nice low shoulders and think, "You're very lucky that I'm here!"' But, if you've got that kind of posture, you do look very strong, even if you're not, and so you can convey that, and it will help you to perform.*

*I give myself a good eye line, too. You want to be looking out and slightly up. When you look out in the RAH, you can see the tiers of the auditorium and there is one that is just perfect. It's just above my natural eye line, so looking at it gives me a long neck, and that helps too, you can't sing properly if you tuck your chin down.*

## Using the body in space

Movement creates drama. When a singer is posturally aware, and adds movement to singing, the effect can be electrifying. On occasion the physical space available for movement is relatively small. You might only have a small area of the stage because of scenery or other characters, or if you are singing a recital, there is still the issue of other players and instruments taking up the space. Neil explains how a performer can use quite a small area of stage to create the impression of considerable movement. For example, simply shifting weight from one leg to the other can make a significant visual drama:

*When I teach people, this skill is simple but vital. For example there's a very static aria that Pamina sings in* The Magic Flute *[by Mozart] that all the sopranos like singing ['Ach, ich fühl's, es ist verschwunden', or 'Ah, I feel it, it has disappeared'], and when they sing it, they tend to sing it all through dead straight.*

*I say to them, 'You can really create the whole world of the stage, the staging you'll be given*

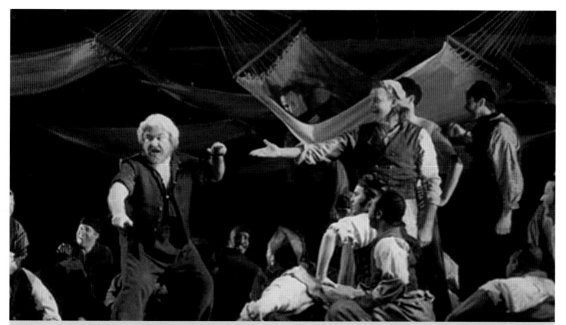

*Neil as Red Whiskers in Britten's* Billy Budd, *Lyric Opera of Chicago. By moving from leg to leg he can create the illusion of dynamic movement while occupying a small physical space. On a crowded set, such as this, there is very little room to move around so this dynamic skill comes into its own*

*when you perform it on the stage. All you need to remember is that you can just shift your weight and you enter a different part of the stage – so you're here [Neil faces forward], and Tamino's over there, and you want to talk to him, so just move – hardly anything, not from your little space – you just put your body onto a different leg, and in so doing it's as if you've said to him "will you answer me?" – but he won't – and then it's as if you say to yourself, "I'm so disappointed", so you change your weight back to the previous leg and look away from him. [Neil demonstrates this sequence of small movements so powerfully, simply standing on one spot, he looks as if he has crossed the entire room and back again.]*

*'So you see I've hardly moved anywhere, but it's as though I've travelled to the other side of the stage, and it's all just through weight shifting. In this way you can create that whole aria and make it so much more real.'*

# Importance of breathing

In order to sing, the breathing has to be extremely free and done properly. If your posture is well organized so your back is lengthened rather than shortened, breathing is much easier:

*I think it [the back lengthening] comes about from breathing properly. Breathing is the essence of singing. You only sing on exhaled air and how the air comes into you and goes out of you is what singing is all about. The individual resonances of air going through the vocal chords is going to make you sound how you sound [your unique voice], but you've got to get the breathing right. And if you do, the back looks quite strong. The difficulty comes when you're in an uncomfortable position [because the role demands it] and having to breathe. I have on many occasions had to lie on the ground and still get the right kind of breath in, so you've got to contrive your position so you can breathe and sing.*

# Singing flat on your back

The days when opera singers walked to the front of the stage, sang their aria and walked off again are long gone. Opera is much more dynamic and lively, and singers are actors as well as singers. If a director thinks something will look better if the singer is flat on their back, that's what the singer has to do. Neil was one of the first singers who had to do this:

*Sometimes a singer has to sing flat on the floor, which is a very revealing thing to have to do because all of your technique has to come into play when you're lying on the floor. There was one occasion when this happened to me in rehearsal by accident and it has made a lot of singers' lives very miserable ever since.*

*I was doing rehearsals for a production of Mozart's Cosi fan Tutte with Kent Opera, directed by Jonathan Miller. It was his first opera production. I played Ferrando and there is a splendid moment in the opera for the two men [who have just successfully pretended to be foreigners and tried to seduce their girlfriends. The women however have none of it and storm off. Then the two men and Don Alfonso have a trio to sing!] So to get into the spirit of this moment, we horsed around and there was a couch as part of the stage furniture. We were pushing each other on and off of it and at the end of our mucking about Jonathan said, 'That's fabulous, it works really well, looks absolutely natural.' Unfortunately, by this point I was lying flat on my back on the floor having been pushed off the couch and then had to sing my big aria 'Un aura amorosa' ['A loving breath']. Jonathan said to me, 'Well that's where you're going to start it.' So that's what I did. It's a big sing at the best of times,*

*but flat on your back it's not easy. But that's what I did. I started the aria flat on my back. There's a point about half way where there's a bit of an orchestral break and the other characters helped me up and I got to my knees and sang the second half on my knees, which was better.*

*Jonathan Miller has produced Cosi in [many] opera houses of the world and tenors come up to me and say, 'Oh, I'm doing Jonathan Miller's Cosi fan Tutte and, do you know what, I have to sing, "Un aura amorosa" lying flat on my back', and I say 'Well I think I can tell you exactly why!' The thing is, you have to find a way of taking in enough breath and supporting it even if you are on your back.*

# An open neck

For any organ or part of the body to work well it needs space, and how you use your body dictates how much space you give yourself. One of F. M. Alexander's discoveries about his voice, indeed his whole body, was exactly that – what you do to yourself affects how well things work. He described it as 'use affects function'. Neil recognizes this very clearly, particularly in relation to the neck:

*You've definitely got to have an open neck. In fact you should feel as if your neck is very exposed. It's almost the feeling you might have if you were presenting your neck to the executioner's axe! The way I think about it is, 'this is my neck and it's got to be very open, I mustn't dig into it and bring my chin down because actually that's going to kink the pipe in the neck' – and if you sing with a kink it makes a different sound – one is restricted and the other is open. So you try not to do that [drop your chin] if at all possible, but you might be playing a character role where you're playing a person who is very humble, so you're a little stooped. It's difficult. You know the sort of sound you want in your voice so you try and find that same sense of ring wherever you are. So I compensate for a difficult position because I know what I want from my voice.*

# Holding music

All concert singers have to read their music. This sounds such a simple thing, but how you do so can affect your balance. Nick commented:

*One of the problems solo concert singers face is holding the copy of the music. If you hold it in both hands, you have to do something that is absolutely wrong, which is bringing the shoulders forwards, and that can also tilt you slightly forwards at the hips. So what I do, and what I tell my pupils to do, is to hold the copy in one hand, as though you don't need it, so it's just there as a reminder. You don't want to be stuck to it, you want to be able to think to yourself, 'I know this work pretty well, but there's a bit there I just want to glance at because somebody's got a lead there and I come in just after that.' Just have the music in one hand so you can keep your shoulders open and wide.*

*Most of the time as a soloist you are sideways on to the conductor, or even slightly in front as well, so you have to rely on peripheral vision for the beat, so you know where to breathe in for the length of phrase you are about to sing.*

# Conducting

As a conductor, Neil is very keen to make sure his singers can always breathe:

*There are a lot of conductors, who, if they have done more work with instrumentalists who don't have to do quite so much preparation before they create sound, don't quite realize that a singer has to put the breath into their body before they can release it into sound. So, the thing I am always aware of when working with solo singers and a choir is to make sure I am showing them [with my hands] precisely how they can take the breath so they come in where I want it. So everything is about the preparatory beat. This means there is no tension.*

*If you [as the singer] have to rush it because you haven't been given the preparation the first thing that happens is you will get tense. So as a conductor I want to give singers time to breathe in properly and also be sure they are placed so they can see the beat. So it's about doing everything you can to take away panic, so they remain calm and can sing.*

# Neil and the Alexander Technique

Many singers, actors and musicians receive Alexander Technique lessons as part of their musical education. The technique is highly valued as a way of preventing injury from poor use, aiding recovery from injury if it does happen, and enhancing performance. Neil came across the Alexander Technique early in his career:

*When I was at the Royal College of Music, we did stage drama as well. Our teacher had done a lot of work with Dr Barlow [a rheumatologist and Alexander Technique teacher, also married to F. M. Alexander's niece Marjory]. Dr Barlow lived a stone's throw from the Royal College in the Albert Hall Mansion, so we were sent to see him. One of my problems when I was learning to be an opera singer was that I had my shoulders up too high.*

*Choir trained people – and up to that point I'd been a choir singer all my life – often have high shoulders, and that usually accompanies the intake of breath, and so that's very bad, and there was tension there. There is tension in some of the ways you are asked to sing – in various church choirs, for example, it's all about tension because it's got to be so beautiful. And I can feel my shoulders coming up now as I remember it. For opera, my shoulders needed to be down. So I needed a lot of help and I was sent across to Dr Barlow. I remember standing in front of the grid he had on the wall and he said, 'Oh yes, you're very unbalanced, your left side is higher than your right and your back's not level.' I felt ghastly about it! But I had lessons and carried on with them for twenty-five years! And it helped me release the tension as it built up in my shoulders and neck, which was my big problem. So that's where I go for help.*

*When I did the title role for Peter Grimes [by Benjamin Britten], a very long, arduous role – Peter Grimes is a very tense person – the whole of my physicality had to create this anger, this frustration with the world, and my body got into some knots. Alexander lessons helped me get through. I felt as if they steamed me out again in between performances. Then when I started to get back pain, I didn't want to go to a physiotherapist because they wanted me to do strange things and they didn't understand the demands on my body made by my profession. I wanted gentle things, which is the Alexander way of retraining the body to get into its right position itself by giving quite gentle commands [directed thinking].*

Neil continues to perform, teach and conduct and still has Alexander lessons to help maintain his balance and posture.

# Chapter 9
# Personal posture stories

## New thinking can lead you to new directions

Posture can have a profound effect on all aspects of your being. Most people try to improve their posture because they want to look better, perhaps to feel easier in their bodies and have greater freedom of movement. Increased confidence and calmness are a bonus. But the subtleties of how you change posture can also change you – and lead to new horizons opening up. If you are no longer constantly nagged by your body and have learned to take the risk of changing something by a mental thought rather than a physical action, you can be led in all sorts of unexpected directions.

Posture is a personal issue. Different people work on their postural habits for very different reasons. For some, posture is a professional challenge; for others it's all about balance. This is a collection of stories from people who have thought deeply about their posture and used the tools described in this book, applying them and adapting them to suit their personal needs precisely. I hope these stories will inspire you on your postural journey.

## Rose, professional violinist

I'm a professional violinist working with one of the London orchestras and the job has many challenges. I typically rehearse for six hours a day with the orchestra and practice for an hour before work. The orchestra tours worldwide so we're often playing concerts the same evening as getting up at 5.30am and travelling halfway across Europe. If the travel arrangements go according to plan we'll have an hour or so to rest in the hotel before a seating rehearsal, but when things go wrong we often find ourselves going straight from airport to concert platform. Back home recording sessions are frequently scheduled for nine hours a day to maximize studio time, and as film scores and commercial music are recorded to a click track we have to wear modified headphones with a heavy can over one ear only. It's a hugely rewarding job but the physical demands are enormous and I can't help laughing when casual acquaintances suggest how 'relaxing' it must be to play classical music for a living.

I first came across the Alexander Technique when I was 16 and at the Purcell School of Music. At the time, although I found the theory interesting, I didn't find the physical benefits particularly noticeable. At that age your body seems to just work and the reason you're playing the violin is because you enjoy it. The Alexander Technique really started to help me when I was completing my studies as a post-graduate at the Royal Academy of Music. By this stage in your career the stakes are considerably higher and the long hours of practice, audition preparation and performance anxiety can all result in unwanted tension creeping into your playing. This was when I really learnt the benefits of slow practice, building up the speed of a passage very gradually while ensuring that my use remained as good as possible. I found that my playing became much more secure and less likely to fall apart under pressure.

It's probably only as a full-time orchestral musician that I've finally got into a regular Alexander Technique habit, by which I mean lying semi-supine (in active rest) most days. One of my routines is 'pushing down walls', as this can be practiced even in a crowded dressing room, when lying down in concert dress isn't an option. Playing the violin is basically an extreme sport and I still get injuries, waking up with a crick in my neck the day after a recording session or developing a ganglion the size of a broad bean on my forearm during a run of *Die Meistersinger* (Wagner's five-hour opera), but I find the recovery time is quicker if I use my Alexander Technique directions. I also support my playing with regular swimming and yoga to build up stamina and improve mobility.

Even after years of lessons I find myself reverting to my tension patterns when I'm sight reading a new and complex piece of music or if I'm in a stressful performance situation, but the Alexander Technique thinking provides a framework to which I can return in repose. My ongoing challenge, which is the same for anyone who uses their hands and arms in an intricate manner, is to support more of the movement from my back. The life of a musician is full of waiting: waiting to play during bars of rest in the music, waiting while the conductor rehearses another section of the orchestra, and waiting in queues for hotel and airport check-ins. At least with the Alexander Technique I've always got something to be thinking about.

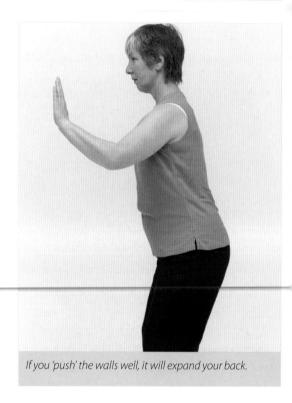

*If you 'push' the walls well, it will expand your back.*

## Rose's 'pushing down the walls' exercise

### Get ready

Each person is different, so you may need to adapt how far you stand from the wall, and how far forward you angle your hips. The main point is to keep your back lengthening so you have proper support for your shoulders. First of all, stand facing the wall, about a foot about from it. Have your feet hip width apart.

Still lengthening and with your breath gently flowing in and out through your nose, ask the big joints of your legs, ankles, knees and hips to unlock, but make sure you don't bend them at this point – just release any tension in them. Are you still breathing?

### Time to move

Now allow your joints to bend so your knees go forwards, out over your toes, and your hips go back, but not too far. You tilt forward at the hips, too, so you are like an anglepoise lamp, but still 'all in one piece'.

Keeping your shoulders wide, bring your hands up, one at a time, and place them flat on the wall in front of you at roughly shoulder height. Keep the sense that your arms are connected to your back.

## Brain and body harmony – the power of thought

This next bit is very exciting but demands a lot of patience and is easily misunderstood. Nevertheless, I think it so useful I am describing it so you can apply your own ideas and thinking to it.

You are going to push the wall away from you! But you are not going to move away from it, nor are you going to tighten to push, or hold your breath. Instead you are going to release your back, legs, shoulders and arms continuously so their increasing length creates the push. The more you apply the twin skills of inhibition (not moving externally) and directions (dynamic internal muscle messages) the more likely it is you will succeed. The experience is one of expanding inside yourself, of your chest opening and your arms feeling strong but supple, elastic and lengthened.

This exercise can help rehabilitate arms damaged by over use of a computer or demanding activities such as those musicians face. Rose uses this exercise to help her stay 'playing fit' in a very demanding career, and you can use it to keep your arms in good condition. If you practice it with some of the other arm and shoulder exercises described in section 2, you will have many tools to help you.

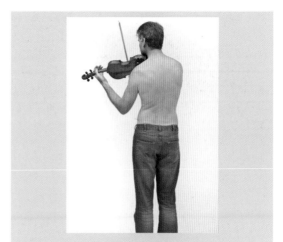

*Richard demonstrates how he used to play. His left shoulder, which supports the violin, is dropped towards his pelvis, resulting in a considerable twist in his waist area. It also increases tension in his neck, shoulder, arm, wrist and hands. The misuse pattern runs right through his body and even his legs are affected. His left leg is rigid as it is propping up his upper body, so he could run into hip problems too. Richard used to play like this before he discovered good use and the Alexander Technique. In summary, he used to pull down in order to play.*

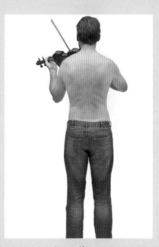

*Richard has generated an effective 'up' support throughout his whole frame. His shoulders are level, offering good support for his violin and freedom for both his bowing and his fingering arm. This freedom saved him from crippling arm and back pain and improved his playing.*

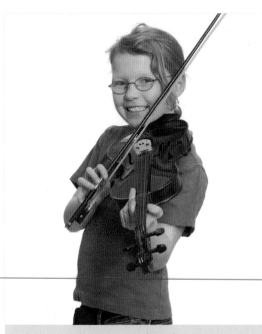

*As Rose pointed out, a young player doesn't notice what the stresses are on their body. This young girl is already demonstrating poor posture and poor body use as she plays. Her back is arched forward and she is leaning back, creating pressure in her lumbar area. This will lead to tension in her diaphragm and encourage her to stiffen in her shoulders. If you look carefully you can tell her shoulders are narrowing in towards the violin, not staying wide and open. She may not feel it now, but playing like this will damage her in the long run.*

# Horse riding without pain – Marie's story of finding balance

I have always been a very active person, I ride daily and look after my horse Gabriel myself, which involves a great deal of physical labour. Gabriel is a 'barefoot' horse, meaning he is unshod and I do not use a bit in his bridle. He doesn't live in a stable, but in a field with a small herd of other horses. I practice natural horsemanship as closely as is feasible in this country. Gabriel doesn't eat oats or any 'heating' foods. To keep a horse like this requires a great deal of effort and dedication, not to mention manual work – which I enjoy. But I had back pain and sciatica, and it was so bad I took over-the-counter pain medication at regular intervals throughout the day, every day. I took the maximum dose and it got me by, but I still had pain and I didn't really want to keep taking pills.

Your back is under considerable demand when you ride. It needs to be strong, but supple. Knowing what I know now, I realize the balance of your head on top of your spine will profoundly influence how springy – or not – you are throughout your back. This in turn affects your arms and legs. If your back is stiff you are likely to have tight arms and legs, leading to stiff wrists and hands. These problems will communicate themselves to your horse; a stiff rider makes a horse stiffen in response. I was aware I was passing on my tension to Gabriel, and I didn't like it. He is such a sensitive horse and I felt I wasn't giving him the best chance to move well, either. I had heard that the Alexander Technique could help riders with their seat and back pain. So I decided to look into it and see if it really could do both those things for me.

After a while I understood the common factor between back pain and good riding was my posture and body use. In the past I had thought of posture as holding my body straight, and held myself up with effort, but now I can see it is a subtle matter, not just a question of sitting up straight or putting your heels down. It's more a matter of how you set about engaging your balance, and it begins well before you get on your horse! I did and still do a lot of working on myself, practicing active rest and thinking about not stiffening my neck as I'm shovelling Gabriel's offerings into a wheelbarrow or carting bales of hay around.

I discovered I had a tendency to lock my head down on my neck. The column of my neck tended to buckle a bit under the pressure, and twist in response – so I was carrying my head on one side. The first thing I did when I was told what was going on in my neck was to straighten it up – but that didn't work – of course! My whole body was compensating for what was going on in my head and neck, and causing problems lower down in my back; no doubt this was the cause of my sciatica and lower back pain. I never thought it was connected to my neck – because that didn't hurt – even though it was stiff. My arms were part of my problem, too. I held them up with my neck instead of allowing my shoulder girdle to sit on my ribcage. It all seemed a big tangle of information to me at first and I didn't know where to start.

Finally, I understood I had to start with the basis of all my movements, which is how I organize myself in response to the stimuli of life – or, to put it more simply, how I cope with the ever present pull of gravity on me. I was going about my day holding tension in my body, and literally shortening myself. This was such a strong habit I didn't notice I was doing it – it had slipped beneath my body–mind radar. Gradually I learned to reconnect with my balance and breathing in a natural way, which gently unfolded long-held tensions.

Over a period of six months I found my pain went, so I no longer needed pain medication. I just stopped taken the tablets because I didn't need them – it was quite a surprise to realize I had 'forgotten' to take them. In the past I'd be counting the hours until my next dose; now I just don't think about them at all. My riding improved enormously and Gabriel is now a very happy horse. My new springy back enables me to respond to his movement freely and without pain. The most fundamental lesson I learnt was how to inhibit my old tension habits from taking over when I rode – or walked, ate my dinner or washed my hair, or carried out any common daily action. It was truly a wake-up call.

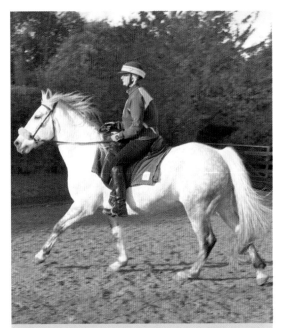

*Marie and Gabriel move freely together. Her neck is free and so is his. He is nicely flexed at the poll, the horse equivalent of our nodding joint. This has been achieved without any pulling on his mouth or pressure on his nostrils. Marie uses a bit-less bridle that is very light.*

# Lisa – pregnant and posturally challenged!

When I was pregnant with my second baby, I knew I wanted lots of help with my posture. My first pregnancy was really uncomfortable. I had constant mild sciatica, considerable digestive discomfort and backache. I was told that my posture was bad and causing compression in my lumbar area, which gave me both back pain and sciatica. It was really bad at times, and although I enjoyed looking forward to the baby, I felt I was struggling all the time. It was difficult to work, too, and I had a lot of time off. I didn't get much sympathy when I was at work, either.

People think you should sail through pregnancy

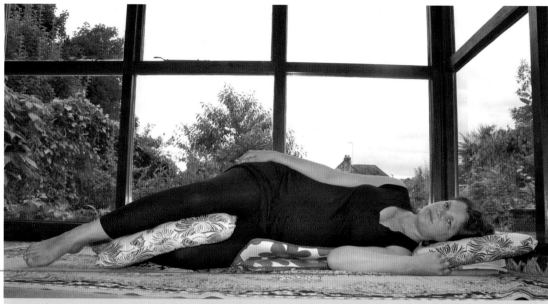

*You can adapt active rest to lie on your side instead of your back. It's still helpful to lie on a firm surface as your body gets a clearer 'spring up' message from a firm surface than a soft one. Pad yourself up wherever you need to by placing a cushion between your thighs and your knees. Lisa is well supported and comfortable. She has enough height under her head to allow her underneath shoulder to release, and enough support under her bump so the weight of the baby doesn't pull on her back.*

with no problems – but I didn't. I wore a supportive corset, which gave me some relief, but I wanted to do more to help myself. My first labour was long, and ended in a forceps delivery; subsequently I felt my pelvis was very unstable and my back pain worse. That was why I went for Alexander lessons. I decided I needed to sort my posture out before having another baby, and then when I became pregnant again sooner than expected I panicked a bit.

As it turned out I got to know my body and posture habits well fairly quickly. The first thing I realized was I had little sense of balance and was very out of touch with my sense of awareness. I went about my days with extreme tension in my neck and jaw. This was the most obvious tension, and a contributing factor to the rounding of my upper back. Friends told me I slumped, but I didn't realize it. Once I became aware of my rounded shoulders, it was also pointed out to

me that the stoop created pressure on my lower back, contributing to my back pain. This same pattern of muscular misuse caused compression in my digestive system and as my first baby grew, everything got more cramped and squashed.

But then I learned to lengthen and as my second pregnancy progressed I maintained a sense of lengthening through my whole body. I loved the feeling of space it gave me. I felt light and could breathe easily, even as I got bigger. I managed to use length down my back to balance my increasing weight and focused on coordinating my head, neck and back in a good relationship rather than as separate bits of myself pulling in different directions.

At seven months pregnant I was very well, with no back pain, and my digestion was working well.

I lie on my side and give my directions now, with cushions to pad me out so nothing is pressing. I have a telephone book underneath the cushion

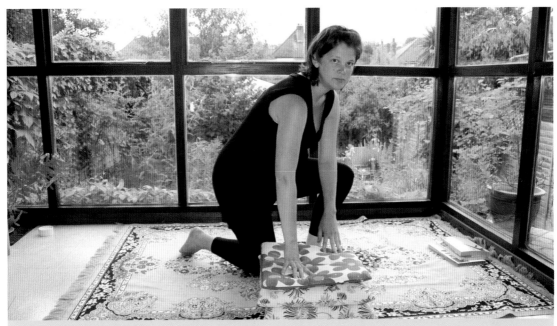

*Get up from active rest without pulling your head back.*

I rest my head on. This gives me support so I can release my neck. I also have a cushion under the bump to support the baby and another between my legs so they don't get stiff. I'm still lying on the floor on a rug and it's really comfortable; sometimes I even doze off in this position, but mostly I feel a gentle surge of energy – it rejuvenates me. I can release through my back and legs; they seem to get longer and longer and I can feel my back breathing and opening. I'm sure the baby likes it when I direct too! Good posture and knowing how to maintain it has made this pregnancy much more comfortable than my last one. When I get up I take my time and do it in stages, keeping a sense of length as I do so.

I find I just want to free my neck all the time – it's so wonderful. It helps me get in and out of the bath, which I remember being a terrible struggle in my first pregnancy. I now realize I was probably stiffening my neck so much with the effort I was making that I was literally stopping myself from moving!

# Francesca's way of seeing

I was never quite the last person to be picked for the netball team at school. I was saved by the girl with asthma, and the girl with weight problems, but I would see the team captains agonizing over which of us would damage their chances least. Now I think of it, it was rather odd, because I was fit and active, spending most of my free time on my bicycle or roller skates, or climbing trees. On the down side, I couldn't run fast or for a long time, and I wore glasses.

Trained by my school years, I learned to consider myself not sporty. So it was almost by accident that I joined the village badminton club, and I was stunned to be picked for the team, not even as a last resort. On a good day (when I had no nerves and for an unimportant match) I could be a useful player, and I loved it. By this time I was wearing contact lenses.

It wasn't until I trained to become a teacher of

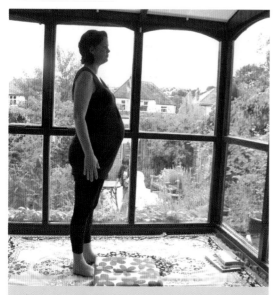

*When you are heavily pregnant, everything wants to drag you forward. Take time to balance well over your feet and keep your back, head and neck coordinated for good posture..*

the Alexander Technique that I put these facts together and wondered. Now that I have got used to wearing glasses again, I notice what it does to me. Of course I want to see clearly, so my eyes look through the middle of my glasses. In order to see something I turn my whole head, not just my eyes. And as my glasses slip down my nose, my gaze goes with them, giving me a habit of looking down. But I am missing out on something in my movement, too.

When the eyes turn to look at something, there is a reflex set up in the strong muscles of the neck to allow the head to turn easily. You can feel this by experimenting. First, look towards one side by just moving your eyes and then turn your head that way. Next, look towards that same side, but turn your head away from where you are looking. You will probably find it is much easier to follow your gaze; in fact, you may have to think about how to turn your head away – it doesn't come easily. Go one step further – close one eye, and then turn your head towards the 'blind' side, and then away

from it. Which is easier?

Professor Raymond Dart says that this particular reflex pattern was probably set down in our ancient fishy ancestry – it was a distinct advantage to turn towards fast moving prey when it was trying to escape.

Now experiment with nodding your head. If you do it without thinking, you will probably find that your sight is fixed on a point straight ahead of you. But what happens if you try to keep your eyes fixed relative to your head, so that your gaze sweeps up and down as you nod your head? It feels as though a lot more effort is involved, particularly in the neck muscles – the head has to be pulled up and down rather than just oscillating quietly on the nodding joint.

If I am keeping my eyes set to the center of my glasses, I will be losing that easy movement of the head to the side, up and down, and perhaps not moving my head very much at all if it is so much bother. That makes me more rigid and inflexible than I want to be.

So how do I go about keeping my head movements flexible? Well, it's a work in progress, but here are some of the things I do. When it is safe to do so, I walk without my glasses on. I enjoy what I can see, and don't strain to make it clearer. When I am wearing glasses, every so often I will look around the edges of them. I will think about the periphery of my vision, blurred though it may be. And I will consciously ask my neck to untighten from time to time – strangely there always seems to be scope for a little freeing up!

# Dai, balance challenge

But that looks impossible! Halfway to England on an overnight flight from Hong Kong, absentmindedly clicking through the entertainment channels, I settled on the documentary *Man on Wire*, for no particular reason. Instantly spellbound, I was watching someone who seemed completely at home in, what seemed to me, utterly unreasonable circumstances. Most impressive to me was watching Phillippe Petit, a French tightrope walker and unicyclist, comfortably 'playing' on a rope in his back garden. Laughing, running, giving piggy backs to his girlfriend – three meters off the ground on a single steel cable. How could that be? Was he super human?

I have a history of participation in what might loosely be described as balance sports. I have experimented with skiing, white-water kayaking, speed-skating, wind-surfing and formation sky-diving. I could perform at a high level in several sports but I did not feel that my balance skill transferred between sports. Rather each sport was a discrete skill developed on its own. I had come to realize that I knew precious little about balance. Indeed my very first Alexander Technique lesson showed me that I had a fairly corrupt sense of myself. In that lesson I felt, and thought, that I was standing balanced and free only to find, with the expert hands of a teacher helping with some accurate feedback, that actually I had all my weight going down through the front of my feet and that I was tensing all manner of muscles and fixing myself to be upright. I probably did that all day and every day! What a relief it was when I settled to being better balanced over my feet, allowing my muscles some respite!

Through life we struggle with balance. Standing on two legs is a bit of a trick, demanding coordination of our senses, muscles and indeed whole body and mind. Generally people are said to have good or bad balance, which we are led to believe diminishes over time. As a youngster you are either in the team or out of the team in school sports. By the time middle or old age comes upon us it is accepted that people struggle with balance. Fear of falling becomes more ingrained, leading folk to become fixed and immovable. Stoops, walking canes and aids become commonplace. More and more of a person's conscious capacity becomes tied up in avoiding falling. In the elderly this can be so profound that one has to wait for the person to sit down somewhere safe before they have the spare capacity to respond to questions or have a conversation. This is something I hope to avoid.

Not long after watching *Man on Wire* I heard a BBC Radio 4 broadcast, which mentioned a slackline – a simple tight rope that fitted in a small bag and could be put up between any handy uprights such as trees, bollards or whatever. I bought one and embarked on a new adventure to explore the questions posed above.

Alexander lessons had been, and indeed were continually, improving the accuracy of the feedback I was getting from my body. I could more readily appreciate when I was tensing un-necessarily, where the bits of my body were in relation to each other and when I was collapsing rather than directing upwards in a useful direction.

Stepping on to the slackline was an immediate and initially overwhelming challenge to my balance. But over time, relying on persistence and good direction from my Alexander experience, the uncontrolled wobbling became calm. Consciously trying not to allow unnecessary tensions to set in and maintaining a positive upward thought or sense of direction allowed my body to figure things out. After a surprisingly short time standing on a half-inch-wide piece of nylon began to feel not only 'reasonable' but completely sensible. A strong sense of a sphere of balance has begun to develop, within which I feel at once free to sway yet remain 'in balance', continually anticipating and correcting, always staying balanced, yet free to move to some other place and a new neutral. I have added further balance challenges, the most extrovert being a unicycle, which I now ride with some success. With those challenges, spread over some three years, I have reached what I see as some very satisfying conclusions. Certainly Phillippe Petit had some very special qualities, but from a balance point of view he was not superhuman. Rather he had spent time finely developing his sense of self and balance. My own sense of myself has changed and become

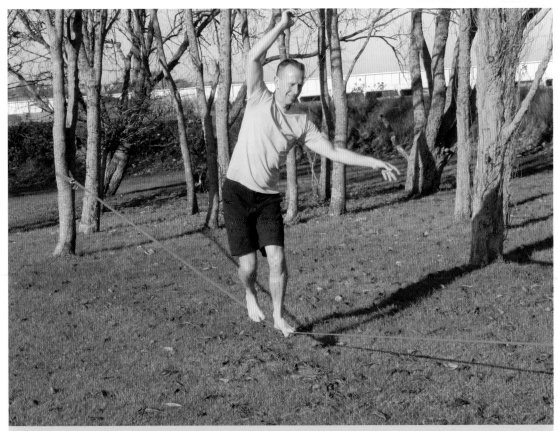

*Balance is an inner harmony of head, neck, back, legs, arms and mind: mind and muscles in coordination. Dai applies the same sequence of thought–posture–movement to all his balance activities. Finally the common factor between all his activities is revealed. It's about him and gravity and it always will be, whatever he does. This doesn't imply that he can do any and everything without practice; skill takes time, but if you have the keys to balance worked out, you will get where you want with less pain and effort.*

more accurate through practicing the Alexander Technique, and my sense of balance has improved dramatically, showing itself in some very surprising ways.

I can now paint around a window frame in strong straight lines, which is very useful in decorating without mess. I am a swing dancer and my dance partners and people watching have independently come up to me and said how much more graceful and balanced I look. I now ski far better than I did when I was skiing 30 weeks a year. As I only get to ski a week or two a year now I find that very rewarding.

My grand and perhaps most profound conclusion, however, is that conscious challenging of one's balance aided by the Alexander Technique can lead to a very positive improvement in one's sense of balance across all life's activities. This is absolutely wonderful. Anyone can do it, and the balance challenges don't need to be as extreme as those I chose.

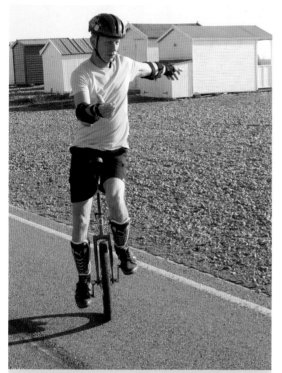

Turning round on a unicycle involves a complex sequence of back and forward movements on the bike and a twisting motion of the body to get round. You can turn, twist, bend forwards, backwards and sideways – whatever you need to do to carry out your chosen activity. If you do this by tightening and shortening muscles you will make everything much harder work. Dai is showing how he maintains a fluid upward flow of muscular coordination through his body, and keeps his neck free from tension. In this way he is able to do whatever he needs to do to keep balanced. It's not about what you do, it's about the way you do it, your inner coordination and your postural unity – or lack thereof. When Dai approaches his chosen task in this way, he brings to it the amount of muscle tone the task requires. What's more, he doesn't need to decide consciously what that tone should be; his coordination, plus the activity, will make it apparent what is required. From there it is a matter of practice. Even if you have good coordination you will need some practice before you can sail off down the path on your unicycle.

# Astrid Holm: posture and creative writing

I've taught Alexander Technique for over ten years now, but it wasn't until I began my MA in creative writing in 2007 that I started to explore the subtlety of its principles in a non-physical context.

To write well creatively, you need to have the oft bandied about term 'an authentic voice'. The Alexander Technique really helped me to develop my writing voice. One of our course books was Marion Milner's brilliant book, *A Life of One's Own*, first published in 1936. She wrote about her journey into creative self-awareness and how she perceived the world in her pursuit of art and self-awareness. The further I read, the more I realized that although she didn't know about the terms 'end-gaining' and 'inhibition', she was writing about her own experience of these Alexander principles. It was fascinating.

I started to apply the principle of non-endgaining to my own writing. A pen and a blank piece of paper is a huge stimulus, not only to drag one forward physically to the page, but to race away mentally, to desire to do it right, to express what you want to say perfectly, immediately… Booker prize here I come!

Of course, the craft of writing, like most things that are worthwhile learning, is a journey. There are layers. It takes time. When reading back a dodgy first draft, I needed to 'inhibit' saying to myself 'this is a load of rubbish' and trust that the 'means-whereby' (involving lots of patient editing) would lead me towards a more skilful expression of what I wanted to say.

Just to have the Alexander awareness to be able to sit and look at the page, to free my neck and breathing, helped take me to a different mental space. Now I really started to enjoy the process of getting from first draft to polished product.

I know many other writers like to meditate or go for a walk to get themselves 'revved up' for a writing session, to make some space in the brain, so the creative mind is free to articulate ideas onto the page. I like to access the mental space you can gain from a walk or a meditation session by practicing Alexander Technique. I free my neck and allow the primary control to lengthen my spine and take me up. This allows what is already there to operate and express itself without interference. Often, it is then the creative ideas can flow.

Having freedom of movement that leads to a flow of creative ideas is a joy in my life. I am able to direct my thoughts towards having the mental freedom to be creative, and trust I can get there, by having a gentle yet steady desire towards my goal, be that a free neck or a poem.

# Dancing with Horace

If you want to help people gain better postural habits you have to be quite sure your own are very conscious and very good. As Alexander teachers we work with people's posture and balance all the time and it's a fascinating but long learning journey. To help someone towards better balance you have to use your hands so freely that you don't impede them in any way, and instead give them a positive direction from your hands. And your hands are only as good as your whole back and postural coordination. So well before Alexander students get to put their hands on real people, they have to learn to dance with Horace.

Horace the skeleton belongs to the Brighton Alexander Technique College. On his wheeled stand he stands over six foot, six inches tall, and he is easily pulled off balance and out of line. He is rather delicate and causes great amusement when he suddenly drops an arm or leg without warning. To wheel Horace across the floor isn't easy. He tends to tip up. However, if you get your own posture well organized, you are connected to the floor even as you move. Then with your hands on Horace, this 'grounding' stimulus is the one you transmit. If you get skilled at it, Horace will glide easily and dance with you.

# Stephanie's story: the joy of overcoming the slouching habit

Newton's third law of motion tells us that everything is supported – ants, elephants, foot bridges and vaulted ceilings of magnificent cathedrals – the same laws of gravity support everything and these laws are universal and constant. Alexander tells us that the human animal is unique in choosing how we are supported. We

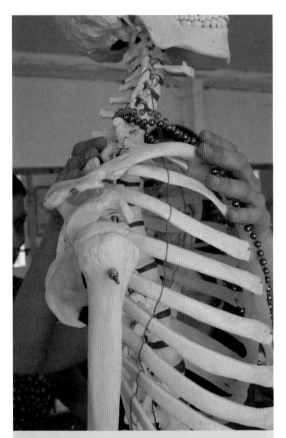

*Horace the skeleton is easily pulled off balance.*

are all subject to the same laws of gravity but we can choose how we are supported. We can choose either to use our support usefully or in ways that are not so useful.

I'm Stephanie Smith and I have been teaching the Alexander Technique in the Epping area of west Essex since 1994. Over the years, all sorts of people have come to me for all sorts of reasons, but they soon discover that posture is the basis of our healthy functioning.

I have always been a slouch; as a child I was always to be found hunched over a book or cramming for exams. I never found things easy, I was always breathless, always tired, and physical activity was difficult for me. I just felt awkward. As I got older, I began to seriously damage my back. After I was completely incapacitated from two major back injuries in a short space of time, friends suggested I take lessons in Alexander Technique. I noticed the difference immediately: I became 'more comfortable in myself', inhabiting my body with a greater freedom and ease than I ever thought possible. I was no longer breathless and felt more coordinated, more in control. I felt that at last I had found something I could do for myself.

I became so fascinated with the whole Alexander Technique process that I decided to train to become a teacher. I became interested in biomechanics and I have introduced biomechanical elements into my teaching. I find it a constant delight to see my pupils grow not only in stature but also in confidence and stamina.

Good posture is everything. It supports us not only physically but mentally and emotionally – you think more clearly, have more energy and just feel good. Vital functions such as breathing, digestion, vision, circulation and so on are supported by our upright posture. For me, the effects of discovering what supports, balances and stabilizes me against the ever-present pull of gravity are unquantifiable.

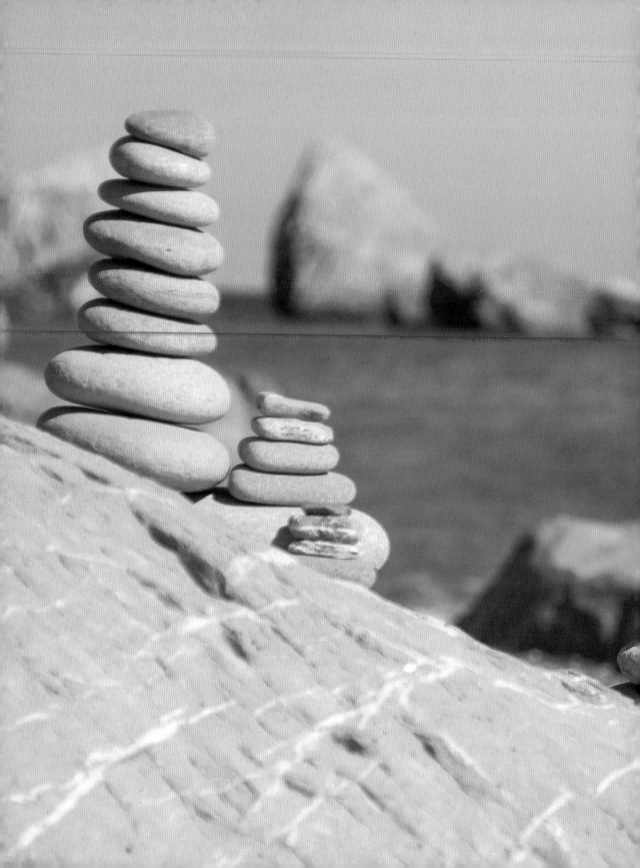

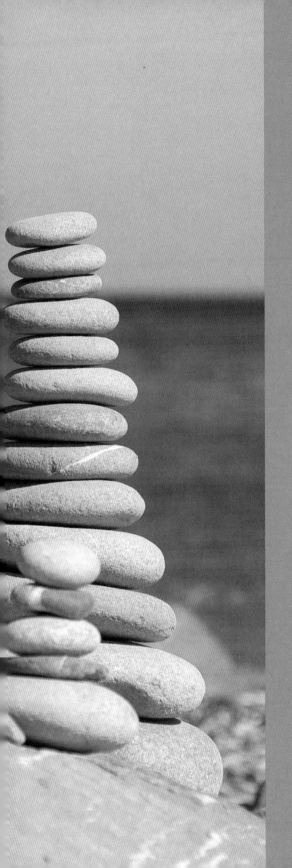

# Section 2

# Specifically designed postural exercises

## Chapter 10
Your postural five-a-day

## Chapter 11
The complete active rest exercises

## Chapter 12
Other exercises for posture and balance

# Chapter 10
# Your postural five-a-day

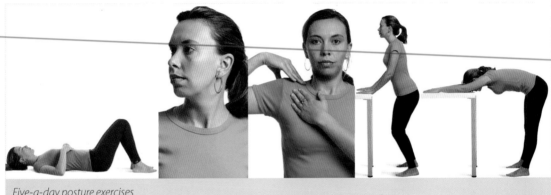

*Five-a-day posture exercises*

I have put together five exercises I consider vital to improve and maintain postural health and mobility. They work together as a group and help you unravel patterns of muscular tension in those places it commonly builds up, such as your neck, shoulders and back. They are all quite simple and can be practiced together as a group or independently of each other. They take between ten and fifteen minutes to complete and I recommend you do them daily.

Don't expect instant changes in your posture; give yourself time to develop the skills you need to do them well. Focus on how you are doing them rather than what you are doing. Take your time to learn each one separately and then put them all together. As well as your five-a-day, I have included many variations, which you can explore whenever you wish.

Your five-a-day are:

- active rest
- head rotation
- shoulder rotation
- body flexion
- right-angled body lengthening

## Getting the best out of this section

These exercises are designed for you to come back to over and over again, particularly active rest, the lynch pin of the whole thing. To get the most from it, keep a journal of your experiments. It can be as detailed as you wish – anything from a few keywords such as 'my back hurt less after active rest today' to mind maps, diagrams or an analysis of the same exercise over time. You can use your journal as a source for reflection, so that if you come across a return of problems you had in the past, you'll have some notes about how you dealt with them. Always date your entries, no matter how brief. It's so useful to see progress over time. There is an example of a diary in chapter 7.

## Silent exercises

Many of these exercises are what I have termed 'silent exercises', reflecting the fact that you make no external movement, usually after getting into a good position. Instead of movement, you are working with the internal dynamics of your muscles, and it all starts at thought level. Remember, thought–posture–movement is always the basis for any exploration you undertake.

A gentle, thoughtful approach to these exercises will be very useful. If you find you don't understand one, just let it be for a while and come back to it later. The patient observer can gain much of benefit in this way. Start with active rest and then dip into other exercises that seem to resonate with you. Each group starts with something simple and builds up into more complex activities. Inevitably, there are crossovers between groups. In the active rest section, for example, there are exercises to explore arms and legs, too. See the table in Chapter 11 (page 128) for brief descriptions, and then find what you want.

## The secret of 'up': your magic red dot

It doesn't matter which exercise you choose; you want a sense of 'up' throughout your body. To help you explore the subtleties of your head–neck–back relationship, which allows that 'up' to take place, you can imagine a magic red dot floating about three feet above your head and slightly in front of you. You couldn't actually see it, even if it was there, but you can aim the back of your head towards it, regardless of your position. By 'aim' I

mean bear it in mind – you don't nod your head towards it or do anything at all – just bear it in mind, that's all.

# 1 Active rest – the subtle art of lying down

Lying down is something we all do. We do it each night when we sleep. In this first vital procedure, we do it to refresh our spine, release excessive tension throughout the body, practice our skills of inhibition and direction, and tune ourselves up! This procedure has various names. I have called it active rest, conscious resting and 'doing nothing intelligently'. I have heard it referred to as 'the Alexander position', or being semi-supine, which describes the set up of the position (on your back, with knees bent). It's more than a position – it's a procedure. Position is half the story, inhibition and direction is the other half. At first you may find your mind wanders when you do this, or you may be bored or think it's a waste of your time. If you can allow yourself the luxury of this time just for you, it will pay you enormous dividends.

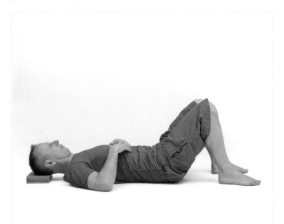

*Lie on floor in active rest.*

This is a gentle but positive approach to human balance, which teaches you to enhance your breathing, co-ordination and movement. Regular practice of active rest allows you to become more aware of your patterns of muscular pulls and tensions, which may be adding to back pain, stress, tiredness or poor posture. It is the subtle art of lying down. Perhaps the most important thing to consider is why you are doing it and what you should avoid. Although people find the whole process relaxing, it isn't a deliberate relaxation; rather you are lying down to become more springy in your body and quietly alert in your mind. You aim to undo habitual tension patterns and help yourself to a better co-ordination of your head, neck and back.

It is the best thing you can do for your posture, back, use and sanity. It is the most constructive 'time out with me' time you can have. Once you understand the basic concepts and are familiar with inhibiting and directing, you can use this procedure to stabilize any back issues, start resolving bad back problems, increase your awareness of your state of neurological arousal, and have choice as to how much effort you are expending. You can experiment with different directions, monitor your improving use and even invent your own directions. You become deeply familiar with your own primary control so it's no longer a theory, but becomes your psycho-physical reality.

## What active rest does for you

Lying on your back in active rest encourages the muscles of the back to coordinate differently and deeply held tensions to start to let go. Your spine is designed as a spring, and the curves help to absorb movement shock as you walk around, and to protect your delicate spinal cord, the highway of information from brain to body. The spine consists of the bony vertebrae (joints) and the softer squishy discs in-between. Everyone knows about discs, especially if they give trouble!

Discs aid the springy effect of the spine and act as spacers between the vertebrae. Because we have so many joints in our spine, we are very flexible, and can bend and twist and more or less move how we want to. The discs are subject to pressure, and as we go through our day our body weight pushes down onto the discs, aided and abetted by gravity. The discs are squashed in such a way that some of their fluid content is squeezed out into surrounding body tissues, and we end the day shorter than when we started. As we get older our discs get stiffer and lose some of their ability to re-hydrate. This is one reason why older people appear to shrink. Fortunately the discs have an osmotic ability to reabsorb fluids when the pressure on them is taken off. One way of relieving this pressure is lying down and going to sleep – that is why we are measurably taller in the mornings – as much as an inch in some cases!

Lying down in active rest not only helps the spine to plump up its cushions again; it also helps you learn not to add to gravity's action by using your whole body with excessive tension so that you are squeezing yourself!

The regular practice of active rest can teach you a great deal about yourself. You have to learn to lie still so you can learn how you move about. This position is a very neutral one. The joints of your arms and legs are more or less at their mid-points of movement range; your back is completely supported and so is your head. You are at rest. It's the ideal place to work on those deep tension patterns, because they are no longer masked by any activity.

When we try to change a basic tension pattern, such as stiffening the neck, when we are doing something demanding, such as playing the piano or driving a car, our attention is always on the activity and our neck stiffening is far down the list of our awareness. In active rest there is nothing to distract you. At first it isn't easy to understand why such an apparently simple procedure can have such a beneficial effect, but gradually you realize that it isn't so simple after all, and what you thought was just about relaxation is actually more complex, and is about your reactions, mental and physical, and that what you are really learning is different ways of responding to the stimuli of life.

## A silent exercise

Active rest is a silent exercise. Once you are in the right position, you don't wriggle or stretch. All change is initiated through the formula thought–posture–movement, although in this case there is only movement when you get into and out of the position.

## First, find your spot

Most people settle for their floor. You can lie on your carpet or rug, with your favourite paperbacks ready to pop under your head. If your floor is concrete it will most likely be cold, so add a duvet or a camping mat. You don't want your feet to slip, so if they do, use a towel or a piece of foam underneath them. It's best to take your shoes off, so your feet can feel the surface of the floor and your ankles are not restricted by your shoes. You can do it on your kitchen table, if it's long enough, or outside under a tree. Anywhere there is a reasonable flat surface that's nice and warm, and quiet so you are not distracted.

## The position – the first half of the story

Active rest is practiced lying on your back, with your knees bent so that your feet are flat on the floor. Your head is raised on a small pile of books so that your neck is suspended between the books and your upper back.

Your elbows are bent so that your hands can lie quietly on your abdomen. You need to consider the following:

- How far away from your buttocks your feet are. Those with a long back might try putting their feet closer to their buttocks than their short-backed friends.
- How far apart your feet are from each

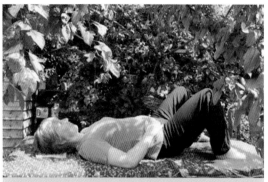

This is my favorite active rest spot, in the garden under the weeping crab-apple tree. Dappled light offers a gentle stimulus to the eyes and the green leafy environment makes lengthening a joy.

other. Generally about hip width – but long-legged people can try having their feet a little wider as this helps them balance their legs more easily.
- How high the pile of books is. This is a tricky consideration. Too few books will make your neck tense and cause your lower back to arch upwards; too many books will press your upper back into the floor (or whatever you are lying on) and depress your breathing. Find your happy medium. Start with a pile about two inches high and experiment from there. More important than height is position. Make sure the books are underneath the back of your head and don't stick into your neck If you have bony bumps on the back of your head place a small folded towel to support the bump. Don't use a cushion as it won't offer the right support.

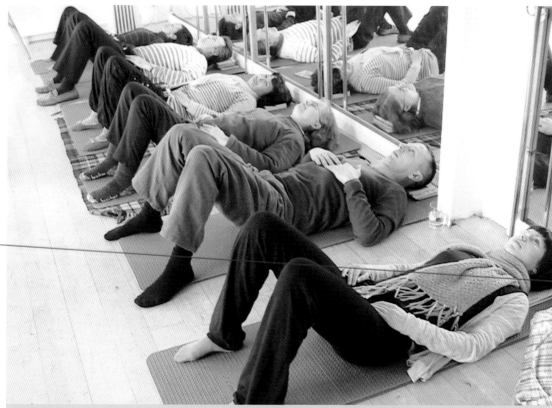

*In this row of active rest devotees, individuals' hands rest in different places, legs are not all at the same position and the height of the book pile varies.*

## Learn to release – the other half of the story

Having got yourself organized the first thought is to come to quiet. If you are a tense or impatient person, you will have a lot of chatter going on in your head. There is no point in trying to silence it; just observe it without judgment and let it diminish. Most mental chatter is associated with physical tension so it's good to notice how the mind quietens when you release physical tension.

### Begin to inhibit and direct
You are going to lengthen your entire torso but not by physical effort or stretching. Instead simply ask your head and tailbone to move away from each other, at the same time. Approach this in

the manner of a request to yourself rather than a demand. Above all, don't try to force it. The key word is allow. This is a broad brush stroke. Now we are going to fill in some details.

### The role of the neck
To facilitate lengthening, ask your neck, all of it, front, back, top, bottom, inside and outside – to be free from tension. Or to put it another way – do nothing with your neck – that implies you might be unwittingly doing something – such as a bit of tightening or stiffening. This will make a prisoner of your head and block your lengthening. To sum it up: *let the neck be free…*

## Head, neck and back

With your lengthening thought still working for you, and your neck nicely freed, you can be more precise about your head direction. With the nodding joint no longer clamped, your head will be able to resume its slight forward rotation as you are no longer retracting it. Taking the pressure off neck vertebrae allows them to lengthen and so the head goes upwards (or if you prefer – outwards – since you are lying down). This release continues down the back so it too can lengthen, and in so doing it too will widen. To sum it up: let the head go forward and up and the back lengthen and widen.

These two phrases come to us directly from F. M. Alexander and are as accurate today as they were when he coined them. You can interpret them in many ways, but the simple truth of the matter is this: if your neck is stiff, you will pull your head back, shorten and narrow your back, and interfere with breathing, respiration and functioning.

## Legs and arms

Your legs want to continue the lengthening direction, so send your knees up to the sky, allowing your feet to stay on the floor, heels moving away from toes, ball of the foot widening from big to little toe. See to it your knees neither fall apart or together but are always tending upwards. Let your armpits widen away from each other so your shoulder joints can be free. This then encourages your upper arms to lengthen out of the shoulder socket, and your lower arm, wrist and hand to continue to 'undo' along their length. To sum up: *direct the limbs to lengthen out of your torso.*

## Getting up

Having gained some release, take your time getting up. The easiest way to do it is to roll onto one side and take it from there. Don't do anything that causes you to hold your breath or stiffen your neck immediately. Having released through your neck, use your head to lead you into upright balance on your two feet. Take a moment to notice your feet resting on the floor, particularly your heels, and then walk off calmly.

## How long should you stay there?

Start with a short period, about five minutes, and gradually build up to about twenty minutes. If you have back pain, it's better to do it little and often. Even one minute will help.

## How often should you do it?

You can't overdose on active rest. You can do it as often as you like and as often as you need. If you vary your approach to it you will not get bored. If you think of it as a task, it won't help you. It can be done first thing in the morning or last thing at night. You can do it when you get home from work or in your lunch hour. If you are about to take part in an activity such as swimming or yoga, you can do it so you start in a good state. If you play an instrument, you can do it before you start practicing, and when you finish too.

## Building skill in active rest

All these directions are an additive thought process rather than a linear one. Basic length is the broad picture you will experience when all the little interferences are released. The detail of neck, head, back, legs and arms is a description of the consequences of that fabulous basic lengthening. They are not a separate side order – they are the main dish!

At first, linking these thoughts together seems almost impossible, but like any other skill you will get better at it. Most people learn to ride a bike or drive a car. When you first start, it needs all your awareness and concentration not to fall off the bike or crash the gears of the car. Like a learner driver, you are going to kangaroo hop your way through these directions for a while. Keep at it – gentle practice will lead you to the one seamless thought – release! And you will know just what it means.

# 2 Head rotation: turning your head with ease

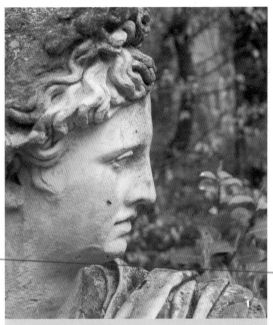

Can you look over your shoulder? Our spine, including our neck, is designed to rotate. This gives us an incredible range of movement. Our neck vertebrae should have a wide range of rotation, flexion and extension movement, so you can turn your head, look up and down, and nod in an almost endless variety of ways. When mobility is compromised for whatever reason, often the neck suffers, and we can suddenly find rotation difficult.

Many people have problems with this movement, particularly as they get older. Reversing the car becomes a challenge. Often it's not age at all – it's bad use! There is an easier way. Essentially, this is rotational movement of the lower neck vertebrae and differentiating your neck from your shoulders. A common misuse pattern is to pull the shoulder and neck towards your nose as you turn. This has the effect of increasing the tension and making the movement more difficult – not less! You can turn your head without over tightening your neck if you think about it.

*You can see the statue retains a long neck, and the chin is neither tucked down on the throat nor tilted upwards. The head turns freely on the axis (the second neck vertebra) and the movement looks natural and effortless. When you turn your head, you want the same smooth action.*

## What to do

1. Sit down, so you can use your sitting bones to get your foundation length up through your whole spine. Then, remind yourself that breathing is always a good option, and direct the shoulder you are turning towards away from you, so your shoulder remains wide and open. Let your nose lead the movement instead of using your neck to pull your head round. Make sure the other shoulder doesn't narrow towards your midline as you do this.

2. Pause a moment and ensure you are still breathing freely in and out of your nose. Then allow your head to turn back to the center so you are looking directly ahead. Then do the

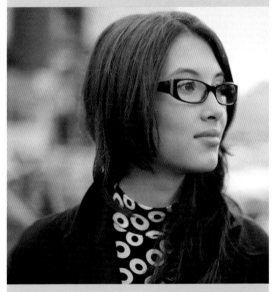

*This young woman is turning her head without tension in her neck or shoulders.*

# 3 Shoulder rotation

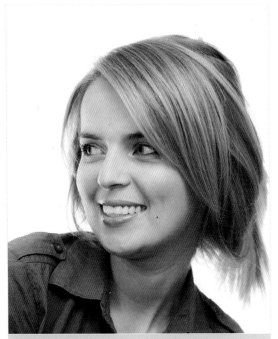

*This is how not to do it! This woman has narrowed her shoulders and pulled them towards her midline. Head rotation carried out like this increases pressure on the neck vertebrae and interferes with free breathing. In turning her head, she has contracted the side of her neck (the side she is turning towards) and pulled that shoulder towards her head.*

We have the ability to rotate outwardly our upper arm at our shoulder joint, but we don't use it very often. It is a vital part of our shoulder freedom but not many daily activities demand this movement. If you turn your palms to the ceiling as you bring your arms up to shoulder height with your elbows straight, then you use this movement – but you won't do that very often! You use it a little in swimming, particularly in back stroke and to a lesser extent in front crawl. It is a vital freedom that is easily lost when most of our activities are carried out with our arms and hands in front of us. This habitual position, which we have to adopt to type at a computer, play the piano, chop veggies or do a host of tasks, encourages us to narrow across the shoulders and also to round them in a little. I wholeheartedly recommend this exercise as an antidote to that. It works best when standing.

## What to do (and what not to do)

1.  Stand freely, in good balance with that lovely lengthening tendency, which should be a part of you now. Do this with one arm at a time, and then if you like you can try both together.
2.  Straighten your elbow and wrist so your fingers are pointing directly at the floor. Your palm should be facing your thigh. Choose which shoulder you want to work with and bring the fingers of your other hand up across your midline, and place them just below your collar bone (clavicle).
3.  Your fingers are now sitting on the outside of some of your chest muscles, which help suspend your arm, and you might feel these muscles start to lengthen under your fingers as you experiment with this exercise. Rotate your whole arm, at the shoulder socket, so the palm faces forward.

same thing turning your head the other way. You might find it helpful to check out your movement in a mirror, but do remember that release is not easy to see so don't aim to make your reflection carry out the perfect movement.

This can seem so easy that you pay no attention to what you are doing. Take your time slowly until you can tell when you are contracting instead of releasing.

123

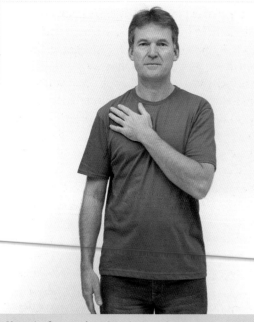

Place the fingers of one hand just under your opposite clavicle.

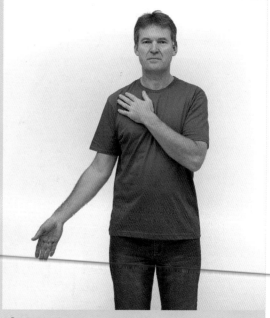

Begin to raise your arm up.

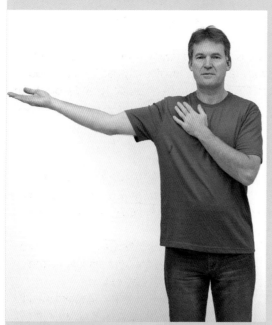

Let your elbow bend.

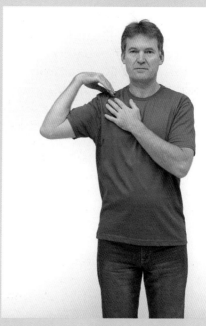

Bring your finger tips to your shoulder.

This sounds so easy doesn't it! But there are pitfalls. First of all the movement should be initiated at the very head of your upper arm bone (humerus), so it rolls in your shoulder socket, and not initiated by your hand, which will always want to lead the movement. Don't let it. Inhibit the hand turning on the wrist or the forearm turning on the elbow. Keep your whole arm in one continuous flowing line. It will come away from your body so that it is about a foot from your thigh. Other tendencies to inhibit are raising your shoulder as you do this, holding your breath, and pinching your shoulder blade backwards. It takes patience to 'find' the neurology to do this movement – but don't give up. You will discover muscles doing things you haven't experienced for some time – if ever. If you are successful, your shoulder blade, instead of hitching up towards your ear, will slide down your back a little and sit on your ribcage almost flat. You are likely to feel this happen. The position your arm finishes in is sometimes referred to as the anatomical position.

4. When you have successfully turned your arm without tightening your biceps, or squeezing your ribs or narrowing your back, raise your arm out to the side, up to shoulder level, continuing to rotate the top of your upper arm so your palm faces the ceiling. See to it there is no tightening in your legs or locking of your knees. Keep your fingers lengthening, and enjoy the widening of your back. Breathe regularly in and out through your nose.

5. Now allow your arm to bend at the elbow and bring your fingers on to your shoulder. If you have a lot of tightening in your forearms you may find this a challenge. With your arm in this position, check you haven't tipped or pulled your head to one side to accommodate your arm. You still want length and breadth throughout your back and legs. Now draw small circles in the air with your elbow joint.

If you hear or feel crunching noises you can be sure this exercise is one you should do daily. Shoulder mobility is vital for good postural health. It affects respiration as well as neck mobility. When you have finished, let your arm float down and hang where it will. If your arms are in bad shape and you find this feels like too much stretch, allow your elbows to bend just a little as you raise your arms; otherwise keep your elbows straight.

You need this mobility for all kinds of things. If you play a stringed instrument, as does Richard, who is demonstrating this exercise, it will make your bowing life easier. Once you have worked out the neurology, which is what takes the time, you can do it with both arms at the same time if you wish. Do it often. I can't recommend it strongly enough. It will help keep your shoulders mobile and your upper back from slouching.

# 4 Body flexion

This is a great companion for active rest, and if you are having a particularly bad back day, you may prefer this to start you off. It can be practiced almost anywhere and doesn't require any special equipment apart from a handy table.

## What to do

1. Stand quietly upright facing a table or a desk. Breathe freely, arms by your sides, taking time to ask for lengthening in yourself and a nice free neck.

2. Ask the joints of your legs, ankles, knees and hips to unlock. At the same time, keep the thought of going up, not subtly collapsing or stiffening, and keep breathing!

3. Allow all the leg joints to bend at the same time so you fold up into a flexed position with your knees bending forwards, and your hips bending back at the same time, a bit like an anglepoise lamp.

4. Rest your hands palm down on the table in

125

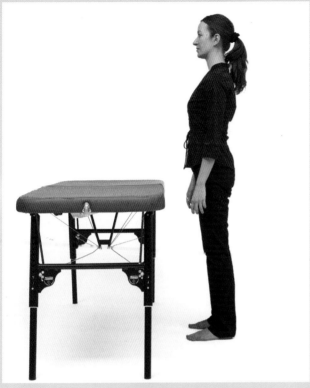

Stand quietly in front of a desk or table.

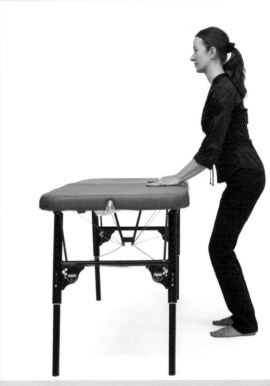

Let your leg joints flex and place your hands on the table.

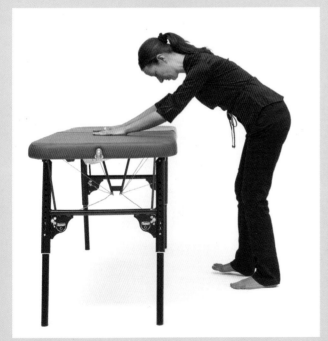

Begin to walk backwards slowly.

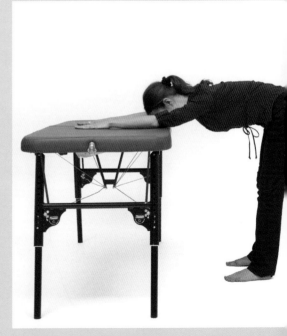

Come to a right-angled position .

front of you (adjust your height by
flexing more if you need to). Keep breathing
freely and easily and stay there as long as you
are comfortable, continuing to ask your back
to lengthen. If you get stiff, come upright and
start again.

# 5 Right-angled body lengthening

This exercise follows on from the body flexion.
Done well it feels wonderful. Things to watch
out for are holding your breath and shoulder
narrowing – you don't want either!

## What to do

From your previous body flexed position walk your
feet slowly backwards until you are at a right angle
at your hip joints. Your back remains straight. You
can gradually straighten your legs if you wish, but
it's not vital and not something to strain for.

# Chapter 11
# The complete active rest exercises

There are many different ways you can practice active rest. It can be used to help rehabilitate a difficult back as well as setting you up for a session of playing a musical instrument or a long session on the computer. Use the table below to help you decide how often and how long to practice.

There are several variations of active rest for you to explore:

- inner expansion
- adapting for pregnancy: lifting a leg without disturbing your pelvis
- exercise for shoulders, arms, wrists and hands
- diagonal directions: thinking about weight bearing

| Your reason for active rest | How long to stay there | How often to do it |
|---|---|---|
| To improve posture | 5 minutes, building to 20 minutes | Once or twice a day – yes every day |
| To ease mild back problems | 5–10 minutes at a time | 2 minutes at first, build up to 5 minutes, then 10 minutes |
| To ease painful back episodes | 2 minutes at first, build up to 5 minutes, then 10 minutes | 2 minutes at first, build up to 5 minutes, then 10 minutes |
| To ease neck pain | 5–10 minutes; add a towel to the books for a little padding | Up to 3 times daily |
| To ease shoulder and arm pain | 5–10 minutes; build up to 20 minutes | Up to 3 times daily |
| To ease wrist or hand problems associated with playing instruments or PlayStation | 5 minutes before playing | Take a 5-minute semi-supine break every half hour of practice; finish with a longer spell |
| To ease hip, leg or foot problems | 10 minutes (legs can take longer to undo tension) | Twice a day or more if you wish |

# Variations of active rest

One of the aims of active rest is to become springier. This will give you a greater sense of space and freedom inside your body. Having gained some experience with active rest you can try the direction experiments described in the steps below. These directions get you in touch with your three-dimensional self. Remember, directions, like inhibition, start at thought level and flow into the body. They don't start in the body (by you doing a sneaky movement) and then jam up the mind. The arrows in the photo below illustrate how you can direct the parts of your body upwards.

## Step 1 Inhibit all interferences

Get into your best active rest attitude and give yourself a moment to inhibit all your interferences and allow some length into yourself. Throughout this experiment keep a gentle flow of thought co-ordinating your head, neck and back, checking you haven't held your breath in your effort to achieve your goal. You want your initial directions to keep going, so that when you add a new direction, you don't completely ignore the directions you have just worked with.

## Step 2 Your sternum

Appreciate your sternum (breast bone); notice it is opposite your spine. Notice its length. Direct the whole length of your sternum up towards the sky. In your mind, create this direction from inside you – underneath your sternum, rather than outside you. Don't worry about your breathing, it will sort itself out; just breathe gently in and out through your nose. Your mouth remains shut. Stay with this direction for a while and enjoy the internal space it gives you. Notice the distance between your spine and your sternum.

## Step 3 Your pubic bone

Appreciate your pubic bone; it is the front of your pelvic girdle. The back of your pelvic girdle is lying on the floor. Just as you did with your sternum, direct your pubic bone up towards the sky, once more from the inside rather than the outside.

## Step 4 Your forehead

Notice your forehead, the 'mask' of your face, your cheek bones and the bridge of your nose. As before, direct these bones up towards the sky,

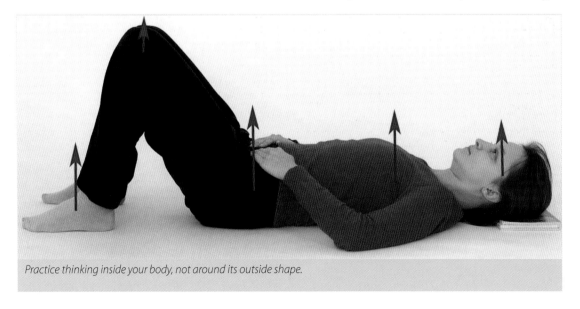

*Practice thinking inside your body, not around its outside shape.*

from the inside of your head. You will need to take extra care to inhibit any temptation to tighten your neck. Take a moment to link these three areas – sternum, pubic bone and forehead – together and ask for the inner upwards direction.

## Step 5 Spreading from your sternum

Let your thinking begin to 'spread' from your sternum to take in the top of your ribcage and clavicles, and the top surface of your arms and shoulder sockets… and spread from your pubis across your groin to your hip sockets. Let the top surface of your feet and thighs direct upwards. Return to the simplicity of lengthening your torso and observe the process of your directions releasing in you. You can stay there for anything up to twenty minutes, but will gain benefit from remaining a shorter time, too. Get up in your own time.

## Lifting a leg without disturbing your pelvis

Once you become familiar with the basics of active rest you can adapt it to suit your needs. For example you can vary the distance between your buttocks and your feet. If you have a long back that is likely to arch in the lumbar area, bring your feet a little closer to your torso. This will make it easier to get genuine release in your lower back. When people have an arch, they are often tempted to tuck their tail bone under so flattening the lower back onto the table. This simply avoids the real issue, which is the lack of good integration down the whole length of the back, and short changes the muscles. Sometimes people do this to reduce pain in that area, much as they do when they let their knees collapse forward when standing to take pressure off their backs. This is an instinctive reaction to pain, and although it may give temporary relief it simply encourages the back muscles to remain either in spasm or lacking in the necessary tone.

When you are lying in active rest, avoid tucking

your tail under. If you have an episode of back pain, experiment with the distance between your buttocks and your feet. This is much more productive than tail bone tucking as it will encourage your back to unlock and start working. Generally, if you bring your feet closer to your buttocks you take the pull off the lumbar area and encourage your pelvis to stabilize.

You can also use this variation as an experimental playground. This is a very useful way to become aware of your own interference patterns around your legs, pelvis and ribcage. The idea is to lift one leg up so the foot is suspended off the floor, and then to extend it so the knee is straight and the leg lies on the ground.

Legs are heavy, and of course strongly attached to your torso! You need quite a lot of tone in your hip flexor muscles to achieve an upright stance that lets you walk. If you watch babies when they first experiment with getting their weight onto their feet, you can see them suddenly fold at the hip joint and sit down with a bump on their bottoms. This is because the hip joints are not yet stable enough to support them. That is only part of the stabilization story, of course. Back muscles and head balance also play a part. Hip joints are a favourite over-tightening spot. It's as if we really want to hang on to our legs. This exercise can help you become aware of the subtle difference between appropriate tone and too much tension.

## Step 1 Your foundation

Get yourself organized in active rest and take some moments to pay attention to your basic inhibition and direction. This will bring you into a nice neutral place. The advantage of semi-supine in this exercise is you don't have to support your back; the ground does that for you. It also gives you feedback. If you do this with too much effort you are likely to notice.

## Step 2 Think of a leg

Mentally select the leg you plan to lift. Does the mere thought set off a reaction in your muscles?

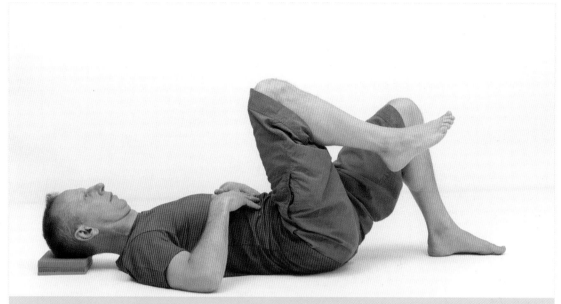

*Lift your leg without effort.*

Can you feel your pelvis tipping towards the leg you have chosen? You are unlikely to do it smoothly the first time – you are much more likely to clench all the muscles round your hips, pelvis and ribs, and probably hold your breath too.

## Step 3 See what happens without pausing first

Go ahead and lift your foot up a few inches, just so you can appreciate all the tightening you are doing. This is what you don't want! Put your foot down and think about it differently.

## Step 4 Will you or won't you?

Experiment at the mental level! Decide to lift your right leg and then give up the idea. Then decide you are going to lift a leg but don't decide which one! These decisions have probably been made with little regard to your basic head and neck balance. I have led you into the 'doing' trap where you are focused on the end result (lifting the leg) and haven't given enough consideration to your process (maintaining coordination between your head, neck and back).

## Step 5 Feel the power of thought

This is the fun bit. Decide to lift a leg – and at the same time, inhibit the reaction of tightening not only leg and hip muscles, but also your neck muscles. Keep a gentle focus on maintaining your basic lengthening direction. Still at thought level, direct your knee to go up to the ceiling and play with making that direction so powerful it (you) actually lifts the leg.

It may take a few experiments before you achieve this – but you will know when you do because your leg will appear to float up of its own accord, with no effort on your part. Still attending to your basic length, allow the leg to extend to the floor. In an Alexander lesson, a teacher will guide you through this movement.

After the exercise go for a short walk and see how much 'holding' you can release in your hips. Don't forget the most important thing – your head direction – without it, releasing the hip joints will make you sink into your legs.

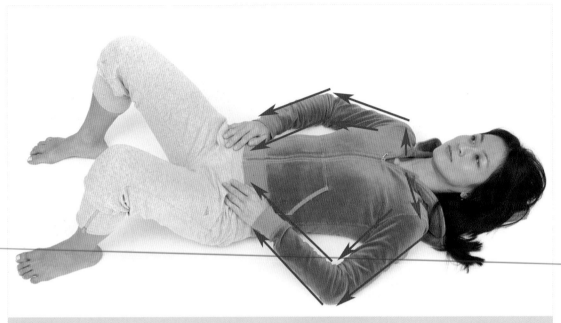

*Learn to direct your arms.*

# Exercise for shoulders, arms, wrists and hands

Directing your arms while lying in active rest is a part of the foundation procedure. If you have problems with your shoulders, or suffer from any repetitive strain in your forearms, wrists and hands, you can highlight your whole shoulder girdle with your directions.

## Step 1 Active rest foundation

Adopt the active rest procedure in your favourite place. Take a moment or two to bring your focus of attention into a quiet and receptive state. Now pay attention to your neck and head directions, asking for length from your head to your knees via your back.

## Step 2 Widen the shoulder girdle

Direct your armpits and shoulder tips to widen away from each other, from the clavicles at the front of your body, and from the junction of the neck and upper back. It's sometimes called the prominent vertebra as it protrudes a little. You can feel it with your fingers quite easily. This is a widening thought, and as with all directions it comes from the inside of you.

## Step 3 Upper arms

Bring your attention to your upper arms and ask them to lengthen from the tips of your shoulders down to the outside of your elbows and from your armpits to the inside 'fold' or 'dip' of your elbow. In this way you are directing both the 'outside' and the 'inside' of your upper arms. Don't rush!

## Step 4 Forearms, wrists and hands

Bring your attention to your elbows, and ask your forearms to lengthen from the whole elbow along both sides of your forearm to your wrists and then on out through to your finger tips. Make sure you

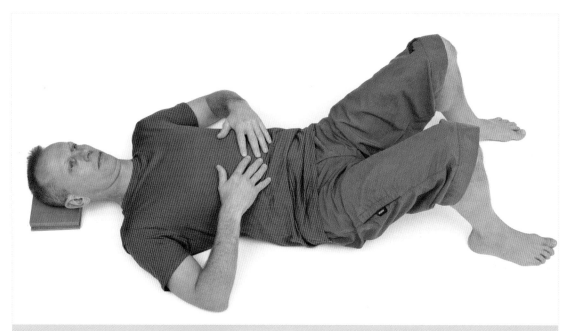

*Lie in active rest.*

keep your breathing gentle, even and constant and you give a spare thought to your neck.

## Step 5 Linking up

Not forgetting your head and neck, direct the whole length of both arms out from your neck and clavicles, blending widening into lengthening, so you link your clavicular dip and the junction of your neck and upper back with your finger tips. Practice carefully and you will get excellent release. You will most likely notice a greater contact of your back on the floor and also a more springy nature of contact.

# Diagonal directions: thinking about weight bearing

In active rest your back and body are weight bearing in a unique way. You can consider several

points throughout your body that are most likely to make contact with the surface you are lying on. This is similar to the inner expansion exercise above, but with the addition of specific contact points to aid your thinking.

After establishing a calm sense of lengthening, consider the points listed below and direct up off them. Take your time over this, particularly when it comes to your feet, which for many of us are extremely tense. These are the points to consider:

- the occiput on the books – the back of your head
- the back of the right scapular
- the back of the left scapular (you may find your shoulder blades feel quite different from each other; don't try and force them to be even)
- the resting side of the right elbow
- the resting side of the left elbow
- the right side of the posterior iliac crest (back of the pelvis)
- the left side of the posterior iliac crest

133

(like your shoulder blades, you may feel
one side of your pelvis lies heavier on
the floor than the other; just observe it
– don't try and force it to change)

- the pad under the right heel
- the pad under the right big toe
- the pad under the right little toe
- the pad under the left heel
- the pad under the left big toe
- the pad under the left little toe

Conclude this exercise by returning your thinking
to your foundation lengthening from head to feet.
This is a great exercise to keep track of over a
period of time, noticing how things change.

# Chapter 12
# Other exercises for posture and balance

These exercises include a variety of ways you can explore posture and good body use. You can use them in addition to your five-a-day and either go through them sequentially or work with any that appeal to you.

As always, what is described is the outer event and what you are focusing on is the inner organization of your muscular support. Remember the principal thought–posture–movement and you won't go too far wrong. Read the description through first and get clear in your mind what the exercise is about. The steps described, most importantly the mental preparation, are all helpful, so don't be tempted to rush.

## Lengthening your back against a wall

The way you stand reflects your coordination. Do you have a nice flowing relationship between your torso and head? Or does your neck droop and your head retract? This is a deceptive experiment in balanced standing. The most important part of it is your attitude. If you are honest about it, you will begin to discover your set pattern of body use, which forms the basis of your posture. This is useful as a marker when things begin to change and improve. Have a notebook beside you to write down your observations. When you come back to this simple experiment your notes will be a

valuable resource. If you remember to date your notes, you'll see your progress over time.

## What to do

Stand with your back close to a wall, but don't lean on it. Have your feet about shoulder width apart, or perhaps a little closer, and stand close enough to the wall so you can come into contact with it (in a moment!) without leaning back too much. For most people this will mean your feet will be about two inches away from the wall. Simply stand there. Don't deliberately try and stand upright or straight. Keep your toes pointing forward, but they don't have to be completely parallel to each other. Stand as normally as you can, looking straight ahead of you. At this point, no bit of you should be touching the wall.

## And then…

Now, very slowly take your whole body back towards the wall, hinging a little at your ankles. It won't be far to go. Which bit of you comes into contact with the wall first? Simply notice and don't judge. You might find it's your shoulder blades and one comes into contact before the other. If your shoulders are very rounded and your upper back stooped you might find your middle back makes the first contact. Just take note of what happens and don't try and change it.

## And then…

Having observed which bit of you makes first

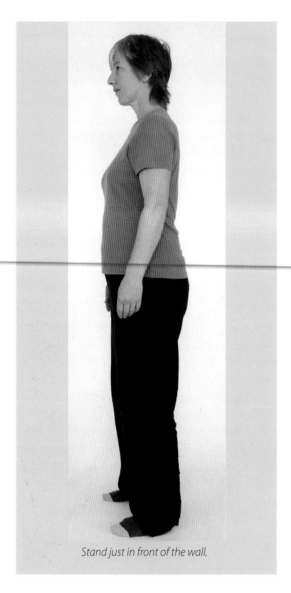

*Stand just in front of the wall.*

## Next

This step is the most important and the easiest to rush. You are not going to do anything, at least not in the way you would normally do something. Instead you are going to direct your body to do something for you. This starts with your thinking. You are going to ask your whole body, from the soles of your feet to the crown of your head, to lengthen. As you do this keep your eyes open and focused, rather than closing them, detaching yourself from your vision by concentrating too hard, or blanking out. Keep breathing gently in and out through your nose.

This is a natural skill of linking mind and muscle, which needs bringing into awareness. The first time you try it you will most likely stretch yourself upwards with effort. This is not what you are after. Be a little patient with yourself and simply think rather than do. This thinking is a direction from your mind to your body. You might consider it a request. If you are the sort of person who finds imagery helpful, think of your head gently brushing the sky and your feet descending into the earth below you – at the same time! What you are after is a simple thought – of lengthening.

Later we will use this thought as a foundation skill to build on, so don't rush it. One problem is the sensations coming back to you from your body. We often use sensation as a way of checking up on our bodies. Sadly, sensations (sensory awareness) are not always a reliable guide, so for the moment put that on one side. If you do notice anything, it may be a subtle sense of your back creeping up the wall as you lengthen. As you walk away from the wall, let your back remember what it was like to sense itself in contact with a surface.

## What happened?

Now your experiment is over, make a few notes for yourself. What bit of you made first contact? You might like to draw a diagram of your body reflecting the contact points. You will then have a record you can see changing over time. Did your toes curl up as you took your body back on your

contact with the wall, very gently continue to bring your whole body back a little on your ankles until more of you is in contact with the wall. You don't need to lean on it, or press into it, just make enough contact so you notice more of your back. Throughout this small movement allow your breath to flow gently in and out through your nose. If you are a habitual mouth breather, make sure your mouth is closed, but your jaw free from clenching.

ankles? Did you experience a sense of fear when asking your body to go backwards? The clues to changing your posture start here. Notice what you notice and don't judge it. There isn't a right or a wrong – there is only your experience.

# Walk with gravity

We hardly ever think about it, but walking demands a great deal of coordination. Head, neck and back must coordinate with each other and with the limbs and head movements. Our posture really has to work for us. We negotiate uneven ground, steps, hills and so on; we manipulate objects such as door handles; we lift weights, such as children, shopping and a variety of objects. All these activities affect our balance over the small platform of our two feet and we must adjust to activities instantly in order to negotiate the world. Many things affect our muscle tone, and if it is inappropriate it affects our walking and all movements. An example is low muscle tone because of alcohol or drug abuse. This clearly leads to failure of walking!

We are going to look at how direction (up) can help us use the minimum effort (muscle tone) needed in order to walk. Walking involves bending at your hips, knees and ankles and transferring weight from one foot to the other. While you do this you have to balance your body above moving joints. Almost any muscle injury interferes with walking, back problems, neck problems and most crucially postural habits. If your unconscious walking habit is to 'pull down' in your torso and you have a back problem or a hip problem then walking becomes a problem.

## Think 'up' first

As always, if you are not thinking 'up', nothing useful will come about. Your magic red dot comes in handy here. So ask for some lengthening throughout your back while you are standing.

## Bend your knee

Then allow one knee to bend so that your heel comes off the ground, but not the ball of your foot. Pause a moment and then release the heel down again, by allowing it to 'drop' with the movement it makes in space – combine movement and direction. Then do the same with the other leg.

Bending a knee sounds so easy! But quite a lot can go wrong. Make sure your hip is not pulled or hitched up towards your ribs as the leg bends, or your body pulled down and across to one side. Let your knee go directly forward so it 'points' over your toes not towards the opposite knee. Ensure you haven't dragged your lower back forwards, which you will if you have forgotten your 'up';

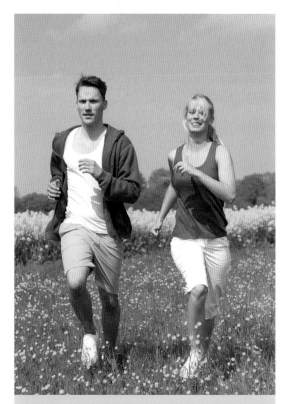

*When your knee bends as you are walking or running make sure it doesn't pull inwards, but goes directly forward over your toes. The woman's pulled in knee is reflected throughout her body. If you look, you will see she is running with a twist in her back.*

finally, don't hold your breath! This knee direction is something you can take into running and you will take a big strain off your back.

## Explore further

When you can lift and return your heels to the ground without interfering with your balance, stiffening your neck, dragging your body forward or holding your breath – and without looking like a zombie – you have made progress! Now try something simple. Take a step forward and transfer your weight onto it. Can you keep your 'up' as you do that? Or has it all gone wrong and you've stiffened your hip joints and slumped into your pelvis? Explore shifting weight around from foot to foot until you are confident you can still 'go up' and move at the same time. It all comes back to inhibition and direction. If you rush you will not notice vital habits. If you inhibit and take your time, you give yourself the mental space to consider change.

## Walk backwards

Walking backwards is not something we normally do, so it can help to give a new experience by taking us out of our usual habits, particularly the habit of pulling your back forward, which makes you narrow and tighten your lower back while walking.

To do this well, you want to take care not to pull your head back as you walk back. Rather keep your head going forward and up, and your knees still pointing forward over your toes. Walking backwards is a good way to encourage your back to stop pulling forward and tightening. This is a good exercise to do after lengthening against the wall, while the memory of the wall is still in your back.

## Go up on your toes

Going up on the toes was something that Alexander did a lot with his pupils. He felt it gave them a feeling of lengthening. It is something you can do badly very easily. But if you do it well, it

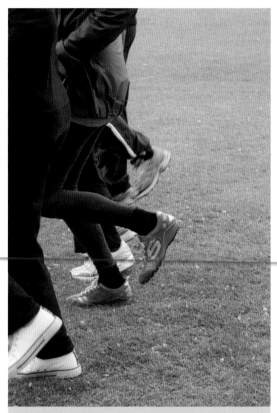

*The ability to lift your foot off the ground without collapsing your knee inwards helps you walk and run smoothly.*

can give you a powerful sense of how you really are one big sheet of muscles from head to foot. A common mistake people make in this activity is swinging their lower body forward in order to 'get up' onto their toes, leaving the top half of their body behind them. This not only causes compression in your lower back, it also suggests the compression is there anyway – and you swinging forward is a result of it – but that is all about to change.

### What to do

Stand quietly, asking for your basic length without effort. Let your arms lie by your sides, with your fingers lengthening. Keep your weight evenly distributed over your feet. This in itself often means

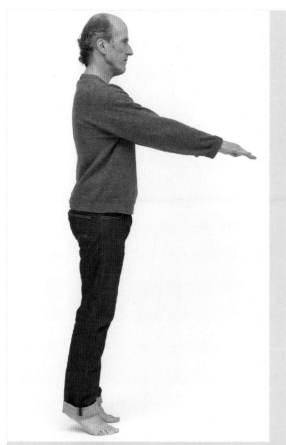 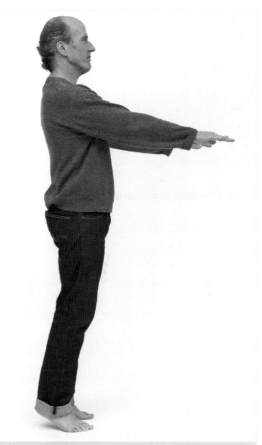

*Can you see the difference between an integrated flow of muscular energy that offers a light easy movement and a movement made with too much effort?*

letting go of a 'forward' pull in your body. This is definitely a moment for your magic red dot. Let your head lead you up onto your toes rather than propel yourself up with your legs. You can raise your arms in front of you if you wish. Ask for length and direction in yourself but make sure you don't stiffen and pull yourself up. Clues will be in your breathing. If you have stiffened, your breath will not flow in and out easily but be held.

# Head and neck directions and movements

Do you know where your head is? Can you tell where your neck ends? Can you turn your head easily to look over your shoulder? These are definitely exercises for remembering the magic red dot. Try them for yourself to see just how much freedom you have:

- Where is your nodding joint?
- Find the base of your neck.
- Turn your head.

There are many elements involved in freeing or releasing your neck, and we will explore some of them. Read Chapter 5 on posture and pain so you have an idea how your head, back and neck coordinate before you try these out.

# First find your head

This is about differentiating the head from the neck. You can try it out sitting in the sort of chair that supports your sitting bones. You are first of all going to locate your atlanto-occipital joint. This is the joint you use to nod your head. In many people it is completely locked and they use vertebrae lower in the neck to move their heads. This makes a lot of pressure build up in the neck. Your head balances on the first neck vertebrae with only a very small area of bony contact, and there is more bony weight in the front of the balance point than behind it. Your head is prevented from just falling forwards by your large, bulky neck muscles. Over use or over tightening of these muscles is part of what we wish to inhibit.

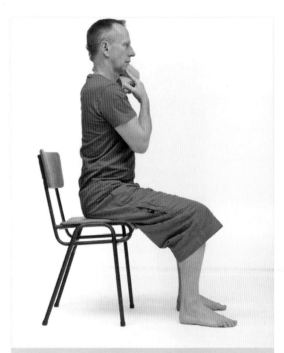

*Put your finger tip in the center of your chin.*

## What to do

Place a finger tip in the center of your chin and gently nod your head forward and back on your nodding joint. Keep the movement very small so you are just nodding your head and not your neck. Take time with this.

## And then

Put another fingertip at the back of your skull, high up under your hairline. Nod again; you should feel the movement of your head at this point. Take time to notice the co-ordination between your two fingertips. Keep breathing gently and don't forget to lengthen up from your seat.

## Next

Now put your fingers on your mastoid process, two bumpy bits right behind your ears. This is part of the base of your skull. Allow your head to nod. This is a movement, and it is easy to do this movement while keeping the joint locked. It takes

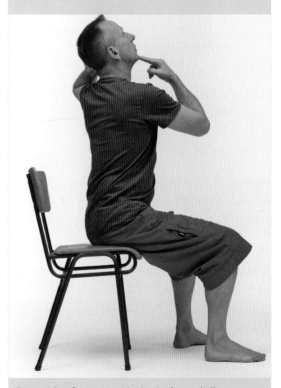

*Put another finger tip at the back of your skull..*

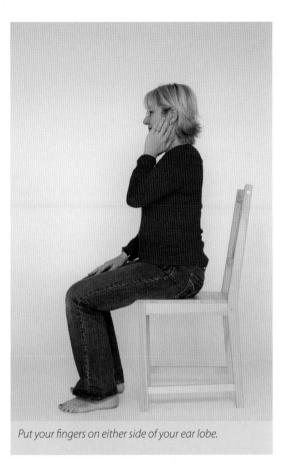

*Put your fingers on either side of your ear lobe.*

head is pushing it there without you realizing it? Consider the angle of the base of your neck. If the whole column of your neck is pulled, or collapsed forward, it will have a negative effect on your breathing and tends to go with your head being pulled back at the nodding joint. All your neck muscles – the big bulky ones you can feel and the delicate tiny ones you can't – need to be considered. If you un-grip your large, bulky neck muscles your neck can lengthen, and therefore your head can go up in space. If at the same time you make sure your 'nodding' joint is free, then the forward element of head rotation is allowed to happen, and – magic! – your head will go 'forward and up' as your neck frees. To help this, try the following silent exercise.

Place a finger tip in the hollow just above your breast bone, and direct a thought, like an arrow, from that point through your neck up to the base of your skull. At the same time direct another thought, from the base of your skull through your head, to emerge at about the middle of your forehead.

time and patience to let the movement take place as a result of release.

## And now

Take your hands away and remake your upward intention, so you are lengthening from your sitting bones. Simply ask your neck to release at the atlanto-occipital joint, as if you were going to nod, but it is a direction, not an action. You might find it helpful to think of the back of your occiput as smiling, or having a breath of fresh air in the nodding joint.

## Exercise for your neck: consider your neck angle

What goes on in your neck? Does it droop forward, or is it pulled forward because your

# Hand, arm and shoulder directions

So many people have problems with their hands or wrists that I have included a variety of ways of 'undoing' tension patterns, including an advanced one at the end of the section. In addition to directing your arms in the semi-supine procedure, there are several ways you can approach this, all aimed at encouraging a good postural harmony so you can prevent tension building up in your arms and undo long-held tension that causes problems.

If you have considerable problems with your hands, these exercises will be of great benefit to you. As I type this, as well as checking my feet are still on the floor and my shoulders where they should be, I take my hands off the keyboard, lay

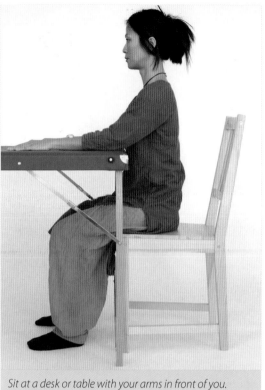

*Sit at a desk or table with your arms in front of you. Spend about ten minutes letting your arms release. Make sure your elbows don't creep up towards your shoulders. This is a good antidote to computer hands.*

it takes any tension out of your neck.

To get the best from this exercise, ensure your elbows rest on the table. This helps you undo the tendency we all have of pulling our arms up into their sockets. Pay attention to directing your index fingers and thumbs forward across the table. You will find in time this direction encourages your whole chest to release and your breathing to flow more easily. It probably won't happen the first time you try it, but with practice you will come to value this exercise for the relief it offers tired shoulders and strained forearms.

Once you understand the releases you can do this as a rest break from computer work. It's especially helpful if you have a long computer session that you can't avoid, but you know from past experience that it will leave you with shoulder, arm or wrist pain. It's always best to avoid long sessions if you can. But if a deadline is looming, you need coping mechanisms and this is one of them.

## Directing your arms and legs to release from your torso

Get set up so you are sitting cross legged on the floor in front of a chair, with its seat facing you. Rest your hands and part of your forearms on the chair.

Ask for your foundation lengthening, from head to tailbone, with your free neck allowing the length to happen. Then ask for widening across your shoulders, and around the six-sided shape formed by your shoulders, upper arms, forearms and the space between your resting hands. What you are doing is releasing throughout your shoulder girdle. Mirror the directions through your pelvic girdle and legs. To do this, ask your hip joints to release away from each other, your thighs to lengthen towards your bent knees, and your lower legs and feet to lengthen towards your toes.

Many people find this kind of release very soothing and you can stay there for a few minutes, or as long as you want. The idea is to release as much as possible without becoming fixated. This procedure encourages your back to support your

them palm down on the table either side of the computer and spend just 30 seconds 'undoing' wrists, palms and fingers. This is a regular habit of mine and lets me type without pain.

## Gentle forearm release

You can start releasing forearm tension in a simple way by sitting at a table and laying your forearms flat on it – pointing forward. Keep your basic length and allow your arms undoing time. Have your hands shoulder-width apart as this encourages the shoulders themselves to begin to open up. Take care not simply to let your arms grow heavy and dead; keep a sense of liveliness in them. Ask your shoulders to widen away from each other so that your chest and upper back stays open. This direction not only helps your shoulders,

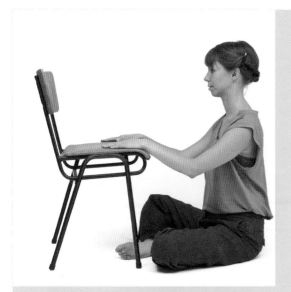

*Sit cross legged on the floor and rest your palms on the seat of the chair.*

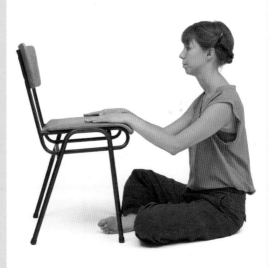

*Make sure you don't let your neck droop in this exercise.*

arms and can be used as a step on from directing your arms in active rest in any rehabilitation program you work out for yourself.

## The lively palm

This is a fascinating exercise, but difficult as it demands a considerable amount of work before you can get the benefit from it. If you try it 'cold' without an understanding of basic directions to your head, neck and back, you will not notice much. But it is so exciting when it works, I hope you will try it out and apply it to everything you use your hands for – from knitting (my latest passion) to holding paint brushes, pens and cutlery, to typing, playing instruments or just holding hands with someone you love. You can try it out in a variety of different ways, so select what suits you.

Either sit with your hands resting palm down on a table, or palm down on your thighs. Sit quietly and ask for your foundation length along your back with a nice free neck. Then follow these instructions, step by careful step. Don't rush it!

1. From your widening back, let your arms lengthen out of your back so you are not holding your breath, and ask your wrists to widen. Think of them like a pair of gates you are opening.

2. Direct your thumb and fingers to lengthen away from your open wrist, through those 'gates' you have just opened. Take that directed 'energy' beyond the physical ends of your fingers as if they were extremely long. Breathe!

3. Gently but clearly direct your thumb and little finger towards each other. You can direct the whole length of the thumb and little finger, or just the tips of these two digits; either works.

4. At the same time, and continuously, inhibit carefully any sense at all of the thumb and finger moving towards each other. This bit is vital, and it sets up a particular and unique dynamic within the hand. You are asking for two apparently contradictory things – your hand widening (because of the wrist) and the outer edges of the hand coming together. Stay with it.

143

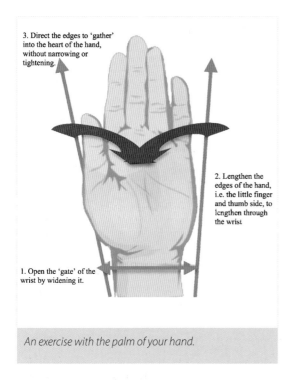

3. Direct the edges to 'gather' into the heart of the hand, without narrowing or tightening.

2. Lengthen the edges of the hand, i.e. the little finger and thumb side, to lengthen through the wrist

1. Open the 'gate' of the wrist by widening it.

*An exercise with the palm of your hand.*

With this combination of inhibiting movement but directing thumb and little finger together… what happens to your hand? You will notice a sense of your palm forming an arch, or a slight dome shape. Your whole hand becomes enlivened and you will make a magnetic or 'sticky' contact between your hand and your thigh. Your palm will feel as if it is breathing or flexing.

Stay with it. As you continue with this process, your hand strongly connects back into your body and engages your back in the activity of simply resting on your thigh.

# Breath and voice work

This is a collection of experiments and exercises looking at breathing and the mysteries of vocal support. Our breathing is strongly influenced by our chosen posture, and in its turn, breathing and voice exercises can help posture to improve. Make sure you read Chapter 6 on posture and breathing before you try these experiments. It

can be very helpful to observe yourself in a mirror while you do them. It will show you what is going on, as opposed to letting you imagine what you believe is going on. Work with a mirror in small doses, and then repeat the exercises without the visual feedback. Ultimately you want to be able to speak, sing, talk, shout or whisper freely and easily without mirrors.

## Open and close your jaw

Sounds really simple doesn't it? But the jaw, neck and nodding joint are so closely packed together that tension in one sets off tension in the other and all tension interferes with the free movement of the jaw.

Opening the jaw is not only used for breathing or speaking, but also for eating, drinking (and occasionally vomiting!). It is a very necessary action that takes place constantly throughout the day. To be able to maintain length through your whole body while opening the jaw is a necessary precursor to the rest of the exercises.

If you wear glasses, remove them for this exercise, as they can interfere with the free movement of your jaw. You might create some subtle stiffening to hold your glasses in place.

### What to do

First of all, allow yourself the luxury of calm, easy release in your neck and gentle length in your body from head to heels, even if you are sitting down. Slowly open and close your jaw several times, dropping your jaw down, away from your head – as if you were yawning. Try opening at different widths. Start with a small opening, go on to 'two fingers' width. Experiment a little.

Ask yourself if your jaw is dropping down away from your head or if you are lifting your head up off your jaw. What does the mirror tell you? Does it match up with what you think you are doing?

## Help your jaw to release

There are several experiments in direction you can use to help your jaw release any unwanted tension

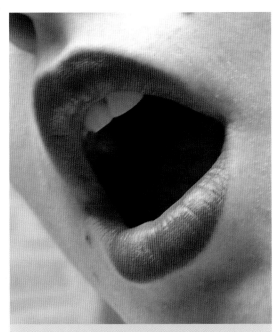

*Let your mouth open freely, without tension.*

directing. Try them out with your mouth closed first and then open. Make sure your first thought is always about your lovely, long, free neck. Try these experiments:

1. ***Back teeth***. Direct your lower back teeth away from your upper back teeth. This can reveal hidden jaw tension right at the hinge. This release can be literally jaw dropping!
2. ***Quiet tongue***. Direct the tip of your tongue to the top of your lower teeth so your tongue lies quietly in your mouth and doesn't add to the tensions.
3. ***Adam's (or Eve's) apple***. You can experience how much the tongue gets in the way if you put your fingertips in the hollow between your Adam's apple and jawbone (in front of the Adam's apple). You should be able to feel the root of your tongue. Having found the right place, experiment with pulling your tongue back from your lower teeth. You will notice and sense your throat hardening under your fingertips. Try

opening your mouth like this. Everything is tense isn't it!

Now once more try out the direction of the tip of your tongue to the top of your lower teeth and open your jaw again. The difference should be very obvious. The message is to keep the tongue quiet, the neck free and the jaw free.

## Your soft palate

The soft palate is part of the inside of your mouth and helps shape sound. It is also part of the inside of your face. Play with making different sounds to see what it does. Each sound requires a different shape. The more you tense your neck and jaw, the harder it is for your mouth, lips, soft palate and tongue to co-ordinate and give you the sound you want.

## Whispered vowels

Try a whispered E, then U, then French U, then Ah. Notice the change in the back of your mouth. This is your soft palate moving as it lifts and widens to make the right shape for the sound you want. Do you remember the English expression 'down in the mouth'? It describes a host of tightness and collapse in facial muscles and soft palate. You can demonstrate this to yourself. Once you know what it is like, you can make sure you don't fall into that habit.

### What to do

Open your mouth and breathe in and out through it. Think really depressed, miserable thoughts and let your face express this feeling by sagging. How does the back of your mouth feel?

Continue to breathe in and out through your mouth and now think happy, bright, cheerful thoughts. Let your whole face express this. How does the back of your mouth feel now? Do you have a sense of it 'raising' or lifting? That is your soft palate lifting. You will feel the opposite of down in the mouth! Having a flexible lifted soft palate will let you speak more freely.

To sum up, to speak freely without effort or pain,

you want an open jaw and throat, but with your facial muscles and soft palate lively.

Having become familiar with some of the earlier exercises, you can progress on to more subtle ones. Remember these are 'silent' exercises, so you ask your body and nervous system to carry them out for you rather than trying to make them happen. Most of them are impossible to 'do', which leaves you a thought initiated direction rather than a physical action. As you think these directions, look in the mirror. If you see yourself frown or your eyes go glazed (or crossed!) you know you are trying to make them happen in some way. Give up! Trying will not make it happen. Stay with directing and if you notice nothing at all just leave it for a while and come back to it. You are rewiring yourself at a delicate level and it takes time.

## Subtle directions to play with

So, here they are. Happy exploring! Work with one set of directions at a time and see what happens. Keep notes in your journal so you can reflect on your progress later. I have called them 'directions suites' to give you the idea that each set of directions comes as a package that works together. I assume that by this stage you understand that stiffening your neck and holding your breath, or pulling down your entire body, is not a good idea! Think postural unity before you attempt these exercises. You can try them out either standing or sitting.

### Direction suite 1
Ask for space inside your mouth and throat. You can break this down into length, width and depth inside your throat and mouth; all are needed for space. Now direct your open neck to go 'back and up'. This is to help you avoid dropping your neck (with your delicate throat inside it). Dropping your neck tends to put pressure on your larynx and vocal mechanisms. Take time and don't predict what results will feel like. Let your body surprise you!

### Direction suite 2
Link your soft palate thinking with your head direction. Send your head and soft palate forward and up together, one following the other; ask for length right up through the deep center of your body, from the soles of your feet right up to your head.

### Direction suite 3
Direct your entire torso 'up' off your pelvic floor. Remember this is thought initiated, not action initiated. This direction will help you not to press down into your abdomen as your breath goes out. Gently blow out through your mouth as you engage this direction. Let your breath return through your nose and gently blow out again. You are aiming to avoid your torso going up and down with your breath. It should remain quietly poised and stable during your breathing cycle.

### Direction suite 4
This final direction suite can open your whole head out if you let it. Once you are familiar with it you can use it to clear your head when you feel 'stupid' from a stuffy room. It can help you clear your sinuses when they get blocked, and make you feel more alert.

Direct from the soles of your feet all the way through your legs, torso and neck and on up through your soft palate, and continue up through the top of your head. Keep this direction flowing while you add on a widening thought by direction up through the top of your eye sockets (under your brows). Let your eyes sit quietly in your eye sockets as you do this. Definitely one for the mirror! Are you frowning and straining to make this happen?

## Explore other sounds and breathing exercises

Different sounds require different actions of tongue, lips and mouth. Play with these exercises and see what they teach you. What they all have in common is encouraging you not to let your breath 'fall' out of your body with no control. If you do this, everything inside you falls down.

## Exercise 1

Make a 'fffffffffff' sound. This creates a narrow passage in your mouth and so your diaphragm, ribs and abdomen adjust slowly to the air leaving your body, and retain tone. This is a good starting point for understanding good muscular support and postural unity when blowing out – which you will definitely want to do if you play any wind or brass instrument – or even just to blow up party balloons.

## Exercise 2

Now go on to try some hissing, just like an angry snake. Put your hands on the sides of your ribs and feel how this stimulates them.

## Exercise 3

This final exercise in the sequence seems the easiest – but it isn't, it's the hardest because it's so easy not to notice how you collapse.

   You are going to sigh, that's all – open your mouth and sigh. Then close your mouth, let the air return to your body through your nose, and repeat the sigh. Do this several times. Your whole mouth and throat are very open when you do this and it's tempting to collapse subtly, but inhibit that tendency and keep your magic 'up' directions working for you, and you will discover a lively bounce in your ribs and back.

# How nicely does your breath flow?

Many of us take little snatch breaths to top up our air, with no awareness that we do it. To see what you do, revert to childhood and get yourself a straw and a glass of water. See if you can produce a gentle, continuous stream of bubbles in your water, by blowing through your straw. If you can do this, it is a sign of having good organization

through your ribs, diaphragm and all your torso muscles. Most of us when we start doing this produce bubbles in fits and starts, like a mini volcano erupting. You are likely to gain control in stages, once you can keep a continuous stream of bubbles then slow it down until you can halve the original speed. When you can do that – you have great control!

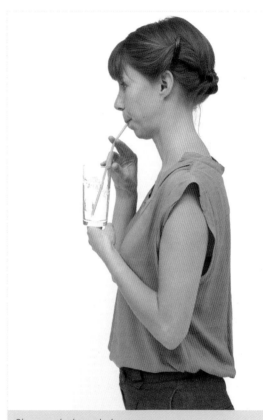

*Blow gently through the straw*

# Glossary

These are some of the terms used in this book and elsewhere in the literature by practioners of the Alexander technique.

| | |
|---|---|
| **Conscious control** | Conscious control is a state of awareness, which is cultivated over time. F. M. Alexander taught that one way of changing how you set about things is to use conscious control. If you are not aware of what you are doing, you are unlikely to change it. |
| **Direction** | When you mentally project a series of impulses (directions) to organize your response to a stimulus according to your choice. For example, to free your neck and send your head forward and up. |
| **End-gaining** | When you focus solely on what you want to achieve, without considering how you get there, you ignore vital opportunities for change to take place. An example of end-gaining is repeatedly bending your kitchen knife trying to put a screw in place instead of getting a screwdriver. You are so keen to get the screw in place you don't think about using a more appropriate method of doing it. This isn't always the best way to proceed. |
| **Faulty sensory awareness** | Your senses are letting you down! If you try and feel things out, you tend to rely on old patterns of use, which lead you astray. An example is when you have spent years holding your head to one side ; it feels right to you, so when you try and change it, the new sensations feel decidedly |

| | wrong. When you first change deeply ingrained habits, don't go with how it feels, go with what you are thinking and asking for. In this way you gradually retrain your senses. |
|---|---|
| **Inhibition** | When you withhold consent to an automatic reaction to a stimulus taking place or say 'no' to old habits. An example of inhibition is when you create a gap in-between receiving a stimulus and responding to it – you stop your neck stiffening and your head retracting as you go to sit in a chair. |
| **Means-whereby** | When you consider how best to get from where you are to where you want to be. So you fetch the screwdriver instead of trying to screw something with a kitchen knife, or you say to yourself, 'I will apply inhibition and direction to this action of washing up I'm about to do – that way I won't end up with neck ache.' |
| **Primary control** | Your basic mechanism for remaining upright and orientating yourself. What is going on in the relationship between your head, neck and spine. It's a subtle and constantly changing relationship, which has little to do with 'straight line posture', and more to do with appropriate tone between the various parts of you in relation to what you do in activity. |
| **Stimulus and response** | In brief, how we know we are alive! Stimulus comes in many forms – hot, cold, pain, pleasure – so many ways it's impossible to count. We need stimulus and respond to it one way or another. We need to understand not to change the stimulus – which often can't be changed – but to change and choose our response to it. |
| **Thinking in activity** | Ah! Nirvana, where you can do whatever you want – any activity, and keep aware of yourself, and your directions, surroundings and responses to the ever-changing stimulus you are receiving. |

| Use | How you use your whole body and mind. Is your use habitually poor or consciously good? You choose! |
|---|---|
| **Use affects function** | How you use your whole self profoundly affects how easily everything inside you works. If you shorten your body, you squash your circulation, digestion and respiration. So how you use yourself affects who you are. |

# Appendix
# F.M Alexander and the Alexander Technique

*It's not about what 'to do', it's about what*
*'not to do'. It's about the subtle elusive*
*art of leaving yourself alone.*

When I first came across the Alexander Technique I was at loss to describe it. My mother was having lessons to help with a severe back problem; she had ankylosing spondylitis, a very painful and limiting arthritic condition mostly affecting the spine. She was stiff, unable to move freely, in a great deal of pain and had to give up her much loved job of primary school teaching. Alexander lessons dramatically changed her life and enabled her to return to work, ride her bicycle again, do the gardening – in short, be as active as she liked. I was intrigued and kept asking her what she did in her lessons – what was this Alexander Technique? Her answers were very vague and unsatisfactory; sometimes she talked about 'thinking tall', sometimes she said it was about not doing certain things. When I asked what these things were she was not supposed to do, she said she wasn't supposed to stiffen her neck, because if she did it interfered with her balance and freedom of movement. This interested me. I didn't see how you could stiffen your neck – surely your neck was stiff all on its own wasn't it, not the result of some action on your part? Perhaps it might be stiff because you had an injury or an illness. Besides, what had her neck to do with it when her problem was in her lower back, where two vertebrae had collapsed? My mother made it clear it was more than just physical considerations; it was to do with the way you thought, which was the precursor to

your movements. Habit played a part in it, she said, and if I really wanted to know more the best thing I could do was have a course of lessons myself. So I did.

Those lessons literally changed my life. I didn't have back pain, and I was an artist, having just completed an art degree in textiles and embroidery. I was busy with exhibiting and teaching and didn't for one minute think I might change course so dramatically. But the lessons changed how I saw almost everything. I felt taller – which as I was already tall seemed odd – and I felt calmer, without ever having been aware of feeling anxious. It seemed to me I could think more clearly, and I could make decisions with more judgment. I was more confident and above all I learned the enormous value of taking my time, not rushing into things.

This concept of taking time has been one of the best gifts the Alexander Technique has given me and I hope it will be a gift for you too. I think it is even more important than ever. We are surrounded with instant access to almost anything we want, and we have become very impatient. We seek to get results quickly and with minimal effort. We are, as F. M. Alexander would have described us, a society of end-gainers, without necessarily considering how it is we gain those ends.

I was fortunate to have been trained by Dilys and Walter Carrington, two wonderful people who were close to F. M. Alexander, the founder of the Alexander Technique, who had a fund of stories and insights about the man and his technique. Walter was of the opinion that Alexander's discoveries were as fundamental to the human condition as those of Einstein. Nicklas Tingbergern thought so highly of Alexander's work that he devoted half the speech of his Nobel prize to describing and praising it. In his day Alexander was widely sought by well-known figures. He numbered among his pupils George Bernard Shaw and Aldous Huxley, who used Alexander's personality as the basis for a character in his novel *Eyeless in Gaza*. Intellectuals, politicians, famous actors and actresses all studied with him and found his methods highly effective. Shaw started his lessons at the age of 80, when he was in poor health and rather frail. Alexander made a new man of him – literally – and Shaw said he felt Alexander had increased the length of his life. As Shaw died aged 94 following a fall from a ladder while pruning trees in his garden, one cannot argue with such a belief. Students would come from America and stay in London hotels purely to have a course of lessons with Alexander. Walter Carrington told me a tale of a grocer who had lessons with Alexander who used to write notes to him, in pencil, on the brown paper bags he wrapped his produce in, sharing the insights the lessons had given him. Sadly, these bags did not survive the passage of time, but Alexander valued them just as much as he valued the praise of the great and the good.

# Alexander the man

The Alexander Technique as we know it today is still based on the insights and discoveries of F. M. Alexander. He was, above all, a practical man who sought practical solutions for life's problems. He himself had vocal problems that were severe enough to affect his chosen career as an actor and reciter. He had enjoyed success in his chosen field up to the point where his voice became unreliable in performance, and despite seeking medical help and voice teachers' advice, his problems got worse. But he wasn't the sort of character to give up on

something he loved, and having spent the first sixteen years of his life in a small community in Tasmania in the mid-1870s he was used to having to deal with his own problems.

In a small isolated homestead, one has to rely on oneself and one's neighbours for everything. This, I think, gave Alexander an intense curiosity about how things – including his body and mind – worked. So he set out to discover exactly what it was that was causing his vocal problems, and soon realized that his problems extended beyond his vocal mechanisms; they ran through his whole body and affected his breathing and movement as well as his voice. They were problems of posture and body use, a big tangle of how he held himself, what he did to his body when he recited, even what patterns of tension were set off by his desire to communicate his monologues.

Initially, Alexander designed a series of experiments in which he set up mirrors around him so he could observe himself when he spoke. He had become convinced that somehow, he himself was causing his problems. This belief proved to be correct and in itself was a milestone of understanding. But Alexander was also a persistent man, another quality of outback life, and despite this initial understanding, he was a long way from discovering all the things we know as the Alexander Technique. His persistence, sheer tenacity and willingness to accept constantly that all his ideas were wrong and had to be rethought from the beginning has given us a series of tools that help us understand our own balance, movements and reactions, habits and awareness. More importantly his discoveries still offer us a deeply effective way of communicating with ourselves, of discovering ourselves and revealing our true nature. You might at this point be asking yourself, what has this to do with posture? If you are, turn the question round the other way and ask what posture has to do with this. The answer is – everything!

# Further information

The following list of contacts will help you discover more about your posture and how the Alexander Technique can help you. This book is accompanied by a website with videos and more information. See www.postureworkbook.com

## Alexander teachers

Carolyn Nicholls (author of this book and *Body, Breath & Being: a new guide to the Alexander Technique*),
www.alexandertechniquebrighton.co.uk

Francesca Aldridge,
www.alexandertechnique-teaching.com

Richard Boland,
https://sites.google.com/site/alexandertechniqueportsmouth/

Astrid Holm,
www.astridholm.com

Janet Jacobs,
www.hovealexandertechnique.co.uk

Sherry Loh,
www.sherryloh.com

## Teachers in England and Ireland
www.stat.org.uk

## Teachers in USA
www.amsatonline.org

## Teacher training
Brighton Alexander Technique College,
www.alexander-technique-college.com

## Photography
www.matthewandrews.co.uk

## Neil Jenkins
www.neiljenkins.com

## Books
F. M. Alexander, *The Use of the Self*
Malcolm Balk and Andrew Shields, *Master the Art of Running*
Carolyn Nicholls, *Body Breath & Being, a new guide to the Alexander Technique*; see also the web link at:
www.youtube.com/playlist?list=PL52264B008203EE2D

# Index

155

# BODY, BREATH & BEING

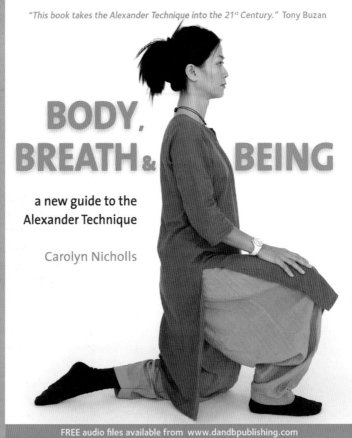

"This book takes the Alexander Technique into the 21st Century." Tony Buzan

BODY,
BREATH & BEING

a new guide to the
Alexander Technique

Carolyn Nicholls

FREE audio files available from www.dandbpublishing.com

# The following are some sample pages from this remarkable book by Carolyn Nicholls

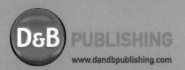

D&B PUBLISHING
www.dandbpublishing.com

# CHAPTER: 8

# Just play the music

## IN THIS CHAPTER

- The challenge of playing
- Why understanding gravity can improve your playing
- Breathing and playing – it's not just for wind and brass players

## Poise in playing

When a musician plays, she or he brings with them not only the knowledge of the music, but all the problems they may have encountered on the way to being able to play that music. They also bring with them something much more fundamental – their relationship with gravity.

The way a musician walks, talks, eats, sits and breathes will largely depend on the way their whole being deals with the downward pull of gravity. And the way she or he deals with gravity will affect the way they play.

This fundamental relationship with gravity is far removed from usual concerns about techniques required for playing, about strengthening weak fingers and interpreting music. Working with – and improving this relationship – can allow the ground to be cleared for a musician to achieve what she wants in the way she wants to, without dictating 'the right way'. Because this relationship is a fundamental that permeates life,

it doesn't have to be practised with an instrument but can be used anywhere, anytime. The best thing any musician can have, and work for – regardless of what instrument they play – is a good back.

## Good Use builds stamina

When a human being is well organised, their response to gravity is one of springy flexibility. Uprightness without effort. Poise. For a musician this is particularly important as rehearsals and performances demand many hours of playing. If your Use is poor, then the longer you play, the worse it will get.

This is not to imply that good Use is only achievable by acquiring the perfect body shape in a nice straight configuration. It doesn't mean that the body parts need to stack up on top of each other like a tower of bricks. It is not that simple. Good Use implies you set about your daily life with the appropriate amount of effort and muscular tone required to do what you want. No more and no less. It is about you as an individual making the best possible use of what structure you have. Most instruments demand both strength and stamina and playing is an all-embracing activity – physical, mental and emotional. Good use encompasses all those elements.

## Woodwind and brass

Any instrument that requires you to bring it up to your mouth brings with it the temptation to pull your face, head and neck down towards the instrument

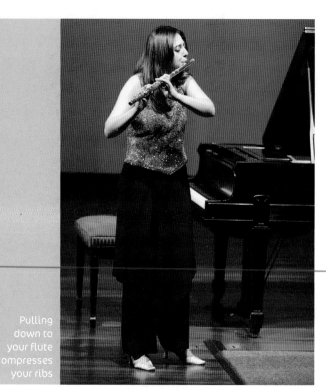

Pulling
down to
your flute
compresses
your ribs

## Mouth to mouthpiece

Bringing your mouth to the flute so you can create a good embouchure is a delicate operation. If you reach forward for the flute with your face then you will simply stiffen your neck and tighten not only your mouth but also your neck and throat – the most likely result being a thin, somewhat breathy sound. Every time you take a breath in you will reinforce this pattern.

## Let your head nod

Your head is heavier at the front than the back, so if you have no tone in your neck your head will nod right forward on to your chest. But if you have just sufficient tone in your neck, and an upward direction through your spine, then you can allow your head to nod on to your waiting flute. This action will stimulate a further lengthening of your back and get your ribs in a good condition to move freely as you play. Your shoulders can stay down away from your ears and your arms are not stiff, so fingers can move easily. This young girl demonstrates good use of her head, neck and arms as she plays.

## Pianists

From the point of view of someone wanting to use their hands, arms and fingers in a complex and intricate way such as playing the piano, good support for the arms is vital. This support can only truly be effective when there is an understanding of how the Use of the whole body, and particularly the back, is involved in the process.

Without useful support, the arms and hands can become both tense and heavy, resulting in a dead, literally heavy-handed sound, that no pianist wants. Attempts to improve this are often made by even more tension that almost holds the hands away from the keys in an attempt to lighten up. This double bind habit is a very difficult one to break. First, excessive tension makes the hands too heavy and then further tension appears to make them unable to produce a resonant enough sound. It's as if the pianist is snatching his hands away from the piano at the same time as putting them on the keys to play.

instead, which will only encourage you to stiffen your ribs and chest. The flute in particular can lure your chin out towards it, thus shortening your neck and dropping your whole neck column downwards. Playing like this encourages a downward pressure on your lungs and diaphragm throughout your breathing cycle. Even if you have learnt circular breathing, this use of your body will strain your neck, shoulders and back. As well as restricting your breathing, you actually make it harder to hold your arms up because you have disturbed your shoulder girdle so much. Your arms will tighten more than they need in order to stabilise themselves and this in turn will make your fingers a little stiffer, making playing a matter of tension. This young flautist has thrust her whole face down onto her flute and distorted her neck. She has pulled down through the front of her body and hunched her shoulders up. All of this will affect the quality of sound she makes as well as contributing to physical discomfort. Her relationship with her flute is uncomfortable.